Pediatric Answers

Pediatric Answers

✦

Answers to Questions You Have Always Wanted to Ask Your Pediatrician But Never Had A Chance to Do So At Your Regular Pediatric Visits

Evet L. Benjamin-Peet, M.D., MBA., MACPE.

iUniverse, Inc.
New York Lincoln Shanghai

Pediatric Answers
Answers to Questions You Have Always Wanted to Ask Your Pediatrician But Never Had A Chance to Do So At Your Regular Pediatric Visits

iUniverse, Inc.

For information address:
iUniverse, Inc.
2021 Pine Lake Road, Suite 100
Lincoln, NE 68512
www.iuniverse.com

ISBN: 0-595-31519-4 (pbk)
ISBN: 0-595-77512-8 (cloth)

Printed in the United States of America

Contents

ABOUT THE DOCTOR

Dr. Evet L. Benjamin-Peet is a graduate of the University of the West Indies, Kingston, Jamaica. She is a highly qualified pediatrician and has kept abreast of the changes in her field not only by subscribing to pediatric journals that are owned and published by the American Academy of Pediatrics, but also by attending Continuing Medical Education conferences (CME) in the United States, the Bahamas and the Caribbean. She has answered pediatric related questions on live radio programs and has also given lectures to medical and nursing students.

Dr. Benjamin-Peet received her MBA for Physician Executives at the Michael Cole's College of Business, Kennesaw State University in Georgia, USA. She graduated with honors in 1999 and was inducted into the Beta Gamma Sigma honors society for outstanding Business Graduates. She is a member of the American College of Physician Executives.

Dr. Benjamin-Peet is acutely aware that patients/parents/caregivers do not usually have the opportunity to get their questions answered in-depth, on a one-on-one basis, at their regular pediatric visits; hence, the creation of this book which is designed to address the social, intellectual, emotional and physical well-being of our children.

The subject matters are arranged alphabetically to facilitate locating specific topics and is presented in a clear and straightforward manner so that a medically trained individual or a novice can understand and relate to the relevant issues. This book is a must read for anyone who is responsible, or may someday, be responsible for the care of children.

This book is dedicated to her two children, Vinette and Alex, who make each day extra special and put the meaning of life into perspective.

INTRODUCTION

The fact that you are even leafing through this book means that you are at least curious about the health and well-being of a child. This book was published just for you. I hope that the material will provide information that will clarify the cause, effect and treatment modalities for each situation and will enlighten you about some issues that you may have been unaware of or have misunderstood in the past. This is not an exhaustive textbook, but a quick handbook for easy reading and on-the-spot reference in relevant situations at home or elsewhere.

ACCIDENT PREVENTION

The vast majority of accidental injuries and deaths in children occur on the road, in the home and at school. For more than a decade, motor vehicle accidents have been and still remain the leading cause of accidental deaths in children and adolescents in the United States. Despite the introduction of drivers' education programs in some public schools in the USA, the incidence of accidents involving teenage drivers has increased. The single most effective deterrent to motor vehicle deaths has been the proper use of seat restraints by both adults and children. The importance of securing a child in the proper manner from the first hospital discharge day cannot be overstressed. A child should never be held in the arms of another individual and most definitely not by the driver while a vehicle is in motion. Children under 12 years of age are much safer riding on the back seat. Infants and small babies should have their car seat facing backward; as they get older they can then ride facing forward. An infant carrier should never be used as a car seat.

It is very important to ensure that the car seat is appropriate for the child's age and weight:

- Infants less than one year of age and weighing up to 17–22 pounds should be placed in infant-only restraints as designed by the manufacturers.

- Infants who are less than one year old but who weigh 20–22 pounds should be placed in convertible restraints and placed in the rear-facing position.

- Toddlers older than one year of age and who are greater than 20 pounds should be placed in convertible restraints in the forward facing position.

- Children weighing more than 40 pounds may be secured by booster seats.

- Children weighing 60 pounds or greater may fit into an adult seat belt, fastening the straps should be done with meticulous care and attention to prevent slipping and unfastening. One should always be aware of the child's position and be on the lookout for the child who will unfasten the snap while being driven. Whenever it is possible there should be someone sitting in the back to attend to the restrained child.

<u>Note Carefully</u>: The manufacturer's instructions must be followed for each restraint system that is used.

Airbags are designed to protect adults and have proven to cause the deaths of several young children who were placed on the front seat of a car. Due to the frequent changes that occur in local laws regulating the use of child restraint systems, it is important to check on the updates within your state. If a car seat has been involved in an accident it should be discarded and replaced, because the plastic may be riddled with microscopic fractures, which will alter the integrity and hence the protective features.

Bicycle injuries also account for a significant number of childhood emergency room visits. It is of paramount importance that bicyclists wear helmets at all times and for increased visibility it is highly recommended that they wear light colors such as yellow or orange and use reflectors and bright lights at nights. They should always consult the local rules and regulations and obey the rules of the road. Whenever possible, there should be a path for bicycles that is separate from the motor vehicle traffic.

Motor scooters, motorbikes and skates also pose a definite threat to this age group and the use of helmets, knee and elbow pads cannot be overstated.

It is important to note that most of the pedestrian injuries and deaths in children are a result of inadequate adult supervision.

Accidents in the home represent a significant portion of injuries in children particularly the 2–3 year age group. The types of injuries vary and range from minor burns to fatal drowning. Most cases of drowning or near drowning occur when the child is left unattended in or near a body of water, for example a bathtub or a swimming pool. This can be as short as the fraction of a minute; therefore it is of the utmost importance that children receive adult supervision at all times. Swimming pools should be completely fenced in and there should be an accompanying self-latching gate.

Needless to say, children spend the major portion of their days in school, from the kindergarten age to the college years and are therefore at risk in these settings. The playground is the site of many injuries, from the pre-schooler to the professional athlete and much more attention needs to be given to this situation. Most playground injuries are related to the surface over which the equipment is installed. Whenever possible, it is recommended that loose sand, wood chips or foam mats be used instead of concrete or asphalt.

ACNE

One of the hazards of growing up is the development of blemishes on the face of a young lady or a young man, during the teen years, when outward appearances play a very important part in their lives. These blemishes are a sign of maturation and are known as acne. They are the result of the action of hormones on certain glands beneath the skin. These glands produce an excessive amount of sebum/oil that forms a good environment for certain bacteria to grow and multiply. The body tries to remove these bacteria and this results in an inflammation of the affected skin, which in turn produces the blemish. Acne may appear in different forms; these include whiteheads or blackheads, bumps with pus, bumps without pus and those that look like large lumps. They may appear as early as 7 years of age and may be present on the face (especially the mid-portion), the chest, the upper back and the upper arms. Both males and females may be affected and cases may be mild, moderate or severe. Some girls notice that they tend to get flare-ups before and during their periods. This may be related to their hormonal imbalances at that time. Although the main problem is coming from the inner part of the skin, quite commonly those individuals who apply heavy grease to their hair and wear a bang tend to have acne on the forehead. This is because the grease blocks the opening of the oil glands therefore causing a build-up of the sebum. Depending on the severity of the lesions, they may heal with temporary redness and darkening of the skin, fine holes, or even permanent scars.

This problem generally gets better with age but there are certain remedies that can be used to control flare-ups and to prevent scarring. The only medication that appears to alter the course of acne if it is used in the early stages, is retinoic acid (isotretinoin/accutane), and initially, it has to be used for at least 4–8 weeks. A doctor, preferably a skin specialist (dermatologist) should supervise anyone who is being treated with this medication. There are some individuals who report that they experience acne flare-ups when they eat certain foods such as chocolates and greasy foods, but this does not happen to everyone. It is advisable to avoid those foods that cause a flare-up, on an individual basis. Certain situations that cause hormonal imbalances in the body may result in flare-ups: these include stressful situations such as physical fatigue, emotional tension or even the cold winter months.

The treatment of acne requires compassion and understanding from the healthcare personnel, because of the emotional impact that it has on these young people and the affected individuals need to have a lot of patience because there is no cure, and control is an ongoing process. The maintenance plan includes gentle cleansing of the skin with a mild soap or in severe cases, using a drying or peeling agent containing sulfur, resorcinol or salicylic acid. This is in combination with a gel containing benzoyl peroxide, retinoic acid or adapalene plus antibiotics such as tetracycline, clindamycin or erythromycin by mouth or applied to the skin. Hormonal imbalances may be corrected with the use of hormones including those found in the oral contraceptive pills.

Acne lesions should not be squeezed or treated roughly in any way because it could make the situation worse. Extremely severe cases may require minor surgery including injections of certain steroids into the lesions or removal of the superficial surface of the skin. Close attention should be placed to the individual's emotional well being and in an effort to boost their self-esteem; young people should be encouraged to base their values on the person they are on the inside rather than on outside appearances.

ALLERGIES

Some individuals react in an abnormal manner to certain substances in the body, resulting in the formation of antibodies, which cause specific cells to release chemicals that result in symptoms referred to as allergic reactions. There is a strong familial relationship among the many different types of allergic reactions. Hence one family member may have asthma while another member may have dermatitis/skin rash. The exact reason why some individuals develop allergic reactions is unknown and although there are different forms of treatment, there is no cure. The most important form of therapy is prevention. Once it is established or suspected that an individual is allergy prone then it is prudent to avoid the common and proven triggers.

Some of the common symptoms include sneezing, coughing, clear watery discharge from the nose, itchy and watery eyes, frequent clearing of the throat and hoarseness due to a post nasal drip, and an itchy skin rash. The more severe cases may present quite suddenly with wheezing and shortness of breath, this could be quite dramatic and frightening. This is an acute emergency because the individual could collapse and die if there is no emergent relief.

Many people have symptoms at different times of the year; this is referred to as seasonal allergies versus perennial allergies which describe those who have symptoms throughout the year. One may be able to determine the cause of the symptoms based on when they occur. If a child develops or shows a worsening of symptoms shortly after being in contact with an animal, such as a house pet, but is relieved when away from home, then one can reasonably assume that the child is allergic to the animal. The major causes of allergies to dust are tiny insects called house dust mites. They live in places such as mattresses, pillows, beddings, carpets, rugs, stuffed toys, upholstered furniture, draperies, curtains and they tend to multiply when the atmosphere is quite humid. Hence although symptoms may occur all through the year, they are usually worse at the end of the summer. Patients, who notice that they show symptoms when they are exposed to freshly cut grass or generally to the outside environment more than when they are indoors with the windows closed, may be allergic to pollen or fungus. If a child coughs or wheezes when he/she exercises, then this suggests that the child may have asthma.

The four main principles of management are avoidance of the provoking agent, medical therapy e.g. Antihistamines, immunotherapy e.g. Skin desensitization and prophylaxis or taking medication to prevent the symptoms prior to exposure.

If skin testing and experience show that there is allergy to dust mites or molds, or pets, then everything should be done to eliminate these sources from the home. House dust mites are difficult to totally eliminate but they may be controlled by measures which include encasing mattresses, box-springs and pillows with airtight, hypoallergenic covers, vacuuming the covered mattresses at least once per week, washing bed linens in hot water (>70 ^{o}C), removing carpets, rugs, stuffed toys and upholstered furniture from the bedroom. Tannic acid or benzyl benzoate may be used to treat carpets if removal is not possible. Vaporizers should be avoided while dehumidifiers should be encouraged, in an effort to decrease the household humidity and hence mite survival. Keeping windows closed and using air conditioners will also decrease the humidity and reduce exposure to pollens and molds. If removal of a pet is not likely, then the animal should be kept outside the house and be bathed more than once per week. An asthmatic attack may be triggered by smoke therefore patients with asthma should avoid exposure to cigarette smoking both at home and in public places.

ASTHMA

Asthma may present in several ways and in the some cases the diagnosis is delayed because there is no obvious wheezing or shortness of breath. Quite commonly, the child may simply have a bothersome cough at nights or when he/she exercises. It is difficult to give a precise definition of asthma, but one may consider it to be repeated episodes of wheezing and or coughing.

There are certain people who are prone to developing asthma and there are certain things such as exercise, cold air, allergies and viruses that will trigger asthmatic attacks. It tends to run in families, especially those with a history of dry, itchy skin rashes and allergies to food, dust, pollens, molds, mites, and cockroaches.

There are three factors operating together that are responsible for this disease. They are an excessive amount of mucus, swelling/inflammation, and spasm of certain tubes in the lungs, that result in narrowing of the air passages. The coughing is the body's attempt to get rid of the mucus and the wheezing is the result of the sound produced as the air that one breathes passes through the narrowed passages.

The best treatment plan is based on relieving all three factors, it must be continuous, prevent or minimize acute attacks and provide excellent control. It is important to note that this is not a curable illness, but it can be controlled and there are instances when a child appears to outgrow the problem.

The primary goal should be to attain complete control and prevent acute attacks. Detecting and avoiding known triggers along with the use of medication may achieve this. Exercise, however should be encouraged, but these children should be given medication prior to physical activity. Complete control means that the child has no symptoms at rest or during physical exercise, enjoys normal activities and has normal airflow rates when tested with a special instrument known as a peak flow meter. There are two main types of medication, those that treat the symptoms of asthma and those that treat the lung inflammation. Almost all children will require some ongoing form of medication; this may include the use of one or a combination of inhalers, liquids or tablets and at times injections. It is important to note that an asthmatic attack may be triggered by smoke, therefore patients with asthma should avoid exposure to cigarette smoking both at home and in public places.

These children require close monitoring by their healthcare professional and there are times when they may need to increase, decrease or even discontinue their therapy. The family plays an integral role in their ongoing care and under-standing, support and encouragement cannot be overstated.

ATHLETE'S FOOT

Although this disease is commoner in athletes, anyone who wears shoes may develop athlete's foot. It is caused by a fungus that lives in warm, moist, dark areas. Sweaty feet that are covered by socks and enclosed in shoes all day long, provide such an environment. Individuals who wear sandals or walk bare-footed most of the time, do not usually get this disease unless they walk bare-footed in contaminated public areas such as shower stalls, swimming pools or steam rooms. This disease is uncommon in young children and is not usually seen before the age of 7 years. It occurs most commonly among preteen and teenage boys. Most cases occur in the summer months when the feet tend to become hot and sweaty, and there is an associated offensive odor that helps to give locker rooms their bad reputation.

The fungus causes cracking and peeling of the skin between and beneath the toes, especially the third to fifth toes. There is usually severe itching and tenderness of the affected areas. If left untreated, it may spread to involve a greater part of the foot, including the nails, the sole (which may develop dry, scaly, thickened patches), the top and the instep portions where the lesions appear as bumps that sometimes progress into blisters that are filled with clear liquid (water blisters) or even pus. The intense itching results in the individual scratching the lesions and this will increase the chances of a secondary bacterial infection, which may result in complications. It may also spread to involve both feet as well as the hand that does the scratching.

Treatment of athlete's foot has to be continued up to one week after the lesions have disappeared. This might mean 4–6 weeks, and even with proper treatment, they may come back. If the condition is not severe and treatment is started early, then the application of an ointment such as clotrimazole (lotrimin, mycelex), miconazole (micatin, monostat), econazole (spectazole), or ketoconazole (nizoral), may be adequate to get rid of the infection. However, those cases that are severe or persistent may need to be treated with griseofulvin (fulcin), a medication that has to be prescribed and taken by mouth.

Preventive measures that keep the feet dry should be encouraged. These include avoiding shoes that provide no ventilation for the feet, wearing cotton socks, thoroughly drying between the toes after bathing, wearing flip-flop sandals in wet, public areas, such as showers, pools and spas, and using an anti-fungal powder, such as zinc undecylenate.

ATTENTION DEFICIT HYPERACTIVITY DISORDER

✦

(ADHD)

As the name suggests, this disorder is associated with more than one type of problem. Affected children are impulsive, restless and have short attention spans. They may or may not have other behavioral or learning disorders along with the ADHD. It is very important to clearly define the specific problems in order to arrive at the correct diagnosis and before starting treatment.

The exact cause of ADHD is unknown but there are genetic and other factors involved that affect the development of the brain before and after birth. The brains of these children are both structurally and functionally different from unaffected children, resulting in their inability to exercise self-control. Boys are usually affected more often than girls are, and the problem is often detected when the child starts attending nursery or pre-school. The initial complaint may be from the teacher who reports that the child is disruptive and disobedient. They tend to get into fights with the other children and have difficulty making friends. They will continue to repeat their offensive actions even after being corrected or punished. Many normal children may exhibit some of the symptoms at any given time, therefore the child has to be thoroughly evaluated by a trained professional in order to avoid misdiagnosing and incorrectly prescribing medication for an unaffected child.

In order to be effective, the treatment plan must involve the family, the physician and the school personnel. It includes a combination of parent training, social skills training, educational interventions and medication. Child psychotherapy can be effective in maintaining or preventing a loss of self-esteem and avoiding social problems. There are instances where the child may be affected enough to require placement in a special education setting. There are a number of alternative treatment approaches available but none of them have been proven to be universally and consistently effective. Support organizations such as children with attention deficit disorders (CHADD) or attention deficit disorders association (ADDA) have been quite successful in helping children and their families to cope with this problem.

There is no cure, but there are several medications that have proven to be beneficial for a significant number of children. Approximately 75% of children respond quite favorably to stimulants such as Ritalin, Dexedrine and Cylert. Medication has its major effect on suppressing the main symptoms, thereby allowing the child to interact better with his/her environment. The child is better able to sit still and listen to the teacher and therefore improves academically. As with any medication, there are associated side effects and these children should be closely monitored.

The more severe childhood cases tend to remain symptomatic in adulthood, but about 50% of affected children appear to function as normal adults. The remaining 50% tend to continue to be inattentive and impulsive and about 50% of this group exhibit delinquency as adolescents and antisocial personality disorder later in life. They may also abuse drugs and alcohol whether or not they were treated with stimulants in childhood. The best outcome is achieved when treatment is sustained and comprehensive, that is, includes special education, parent counseling, medication and psychotherapy.

BACTERIAL MENINGITIS

Meningitis is one of the most serious illnesses that may occur in anyone's life-time, but with early diagnosis and advances in the treatment, only a minority of cases is associated with significant complications or long lasting effects. Bacteria may enter the blood stream from an area of infection, such as the throat and then lodge in the area around the brain, where they multiply and produce an inflammatory reaction that causes swelling of the material covering the brain (meninges). This swelling causes increased pressure on the brain with stretching of the blood vessels and other related structures, resulting in a headache and other symptoms including: vomiting, blurred vision, weakness, irritability, lack of appetite, stiffness of the neck, difficulty walking and in severe cases there may be seizures, coma and death. The soft spot or mole at the top of an infant's head (fontanel) may appear quite full or bulging as a result of the increased pressure. Although most of these ill children will have a high fever (> 102° F), there have been cases where a child had only a mild fever or none at all.

Meningitis may occur at any age, and before the 1990's the Haemophilus Influenzae bacteria was responsible for approximately 70% of cases in children. However, due to the routine immunization of children between the ages of 2 months and 5 years, with the H. Influenzae type B vaccine, there has been a dramatic decrease in the incidence of meningitis caused by this organism. Many organisms including bacteria, viruses and parasites may cause meningitis, but pneumococcus and meningococcus are the two main bacteria that now cause meningitis in children. Infections are transmitted via secretions from the nose or throat and can occur at any time of the year, but outbreaks are more common during the winter and spring months when cough and colds are at their peak. Most infections are acquired from a contact in a daycare center, an ill patient or an adult family member who is not ill, but has the bacteria in the back of his/her throat.

The management of meningitis involves hospitalization of the child, taking blood samples, taking fluid from the spine, performing several laboratory investigations and in a few cases a CT (Computerized Tomography) or MRI (Magnetic Resonance Imaging) scan of the brain may be necessary. The child will receive antibiotics for about 7–10 days but sometimes up to 3 weeks depending on the organism and whether or not there are any complications. The commonest problem following an episode of meningitis, is some degree of hearing loss and less common but significant ones include mental retardation, seizures, delayed language development, visual difficulties and behavioral problems. All children who have had meningitis should undergo hearing tests before and after discharge from hospital and repeated follow up for those found to have any degree of hearing loss. With early recognition, diagnosis and treatment, most patients recover and remain healthy with normal growth and development.

Having meningitis does not result in developing immunity to another attack, but vaccines and antibiotics given to susceptible individuals and high-risk contacts have decreased the number and severity of some cases of meningitis.

BATHING THE NEWBORN INFANT

Many parents are wary about bathing their newborn infant because of fear of wetting the umbilical cord, but if one recalls that the child was suspended in fluid in the womb this may help to allay some of the fear and anxiety.

The clamping of the cord prevents any communication between the outside world and inside the infant. Therefore there is no reason why a term newborn infant should not be given a bath. One should use a mild soap and if the infant has dry skin then unscented baby oil may be added to the water.

It is of paramount importance that the infant is held in a manner that prevents slipping. The best position is achieved by gripping the infant by the underarm areas. The hair can also be shampooed at bath time. The frequency of the baths may vary but I recommend daily baths.

An infant should never be left unattended in or near a body of water regardless of the amount, because this age group is prone to drowning in a very small amount of water. Bath time can be a significant bonding experience and should not be viewed as a chore that should be rushed through as quickly as possible. The baby should be allowed to enjoy the feel of the water and as he or she grows, be allowed to splash and play in the water. Remember that this is the environment that they were accustomed to for the first months of their lives.

BEDWETTING

◆

(ENURESIS)

Bedwetting may be present in as much as 10 % of normal 5 year old and 1 % of normal 15 year old children. It tends to run in families and it is more common in boys and first-born children.

There are two different forms of bedwetting: the persistent type, where the child has never been able to control his bladder and the regressive type, where a child who was trained in this regard now starts to wet the bed again.

The persistent type is most often due to inadequate or inappropriate training experiences or may be secondary to chronic psychologic stress that is totally unrelated to toilet training. In a few instances a serious underlying problem affecting the nervous system may prevent the child from exercising voluntary control over his/her bladder function.

The regressive type is usually associated with a stressful occurrence such as the birth of a new sibling, a move to a new home, marital problems, or death in the family. In these situations bedwetting often occurs on and off and is a short-lived problem. In rare instances, this type may also be associated with a serious underlying problem affecting the nervous system.

In both cases, the child should be seen and evaluated by a healthcare professional to determine the cause and to formulate a treatment plan. The most basic approach would be to perform a thorough physical examination and test the child's urine for evidence of an infection, diabetes or other problems that may cause such a symptom. Depending on the findings, the child may or may not need any further investigations. Treatment varies, depending on the cause of the problem. Several motivating techniques have been successful with some children whilst others require more intense intervention such as conditioning with a mechanical device that rings when it gets wet or even the use of medication. A few of the general suggestions include:

- Using a star chart and rewarding the child for being dry at nights. The reward should be increased as the number of dry nights increase.

- Withholding liquids after dinnertime.

- Emptying the bladder before going to bed.

- Allowing the older child to launder his/her own pajamas and bed linen.

- Praising the child for dry nights while refraining from humiliating or punishing him/her for wet nights.

- Bladder strengthening exercises.

The most important thing to remember is that if the child is given time, patience and encouragement he/she will be successful and maintain an intact self-esteem.

BEHAVIOR PROBLEMS

Everyone has heard the term, "The Terrible Twos." However, if one realizes that between the ages of 2–3 years, children are at a stage where they develop a need to be in charge of situations and to have things done their way, then one will begin to understand why they behave the way they do. At this age they usually lack the social and motor skills required to be successful in their desire for control and this results in frustration and anger. Many of them will resort to crying, screaming, holding their breaths for long periods, temper tantrums and even throwing objects, hitting or biting others. As they get older they may act out by resorting to stealing, lying and even becoming "accident-prone."

At any stage, they are seeking parental intervention or attention and it is the parent's job to ensure that they guide them in the correct manner in order to achieve positive results. It is important to praise children who are successful in controlling anger, but not to ridicule them when they fail, because they internalize negative views of themselves while they thrive on praise. Parents should offer guidance and support to their children, which will result in a feeling of security and high self-esteem.

Children often learn by example, therefore parents have to be careful about the way they manage themselves in vexing situations. It is also important to teach them that it is okay to express anger, but they have to be guided in such a way that they do so in an acceptable and appropriate manner. As a matter of fact they are usually quite scared of their own feelings and the reactions that they sometimes receive from their parents.

A very effective method of dealing with such situations involve giving the child acceptable choices. This provides options and reassurance for him or her, resulting in a feeling of accomplishment and security. Always remember to be consistent, gentle and firm in the management of these situations and if the child becomes uncontrollable and irrational, simply ensure that he or she is not at risk of bodily harm and then walk away until the episode subsides. Children must be allowed to express themselves and be made to realize that it is normal to be angry, but they will also have to learn how to control intensely angry feelings, because this is a part of growing up and becoming socially accepted.

BREASTFEEDING

A mother's milk is by far the best source of nutrition for a full term infant and the practice of breastfeeding should be encouraged whenever it is at all possible. It is best to start breastfeeding shortly after delivery and then allow the infant to feed on demand unless there are reasons not to do so. Although most of their nourishment is obtained in the first 5 minutes of sucking, most babies will feed for 20–30 minutes, every 2–3 hours around the clock. Some babies tend to have a preference for feeding on one breast over the other, but it is a good idea to share the feed time between both breasts in order to prevent engorgement and over enlargement of one breast compared to the other. Retracted nipples (sunken inwards) might make breastfeeding a bit more difficult but it is not impossible. The assistance of a knowledgeable volunteer such as one from the La Leche league international, or a healthcare assistant may be beneficial. If for any reason, it is not possible for the mother to breastfeed then she may be encouraged to pump the milk from the breast and offer it to the baby from a bottle. Breast milk may be stored in the refrigerator for 24 hours and as long as 1 month if it is frozen. It is recommended that babies should be breastfed for the first 6–12 months of life. Although the iron in breast milk is easily absorbed, the infant is born with enough iron stores to last for only about 6 months and will therefore need supplementation to satisfy the requirements of the rapidly growing baby. A cereal containing iron should be added to the diet between 4–6 months of age.

Formula fed babies may gain weight and grow just as well as the breast fed ones, but there are certain advantages that breastfeeding have over formula feeding. Included among these are:

- Protection against infections, such as pneumonia, meningitis, ear infections, vomiting and diarrhea (gastro-enteritis).

- Protection against allergies and intolerance to cow's milk.

- Readily available. There is no need to warm it up or to cool it down because the temperature is always right.

- It is sterile and there is no risk of contamination because of improper storage or preparation.

- It is inexpensive. Lack of funds does not place the baby at risk of hunger and malnutrition. The mother needs to have a well balanced diet but the baby will thrive at the mother's expense even if she is not eating adequately.

- It helps the mother to get back into shape faster than if she were not breastfeeding, because the sucking of the baby triggers the release of a hormone that causes the uterus to contract and consequently allows the abdomen to become smaller.

- It hastens weight loss in the mother because the production of milk results in the burning of calories. The mother can therefore eat a well balanced diet and still lose weight while she is breastfeeding.

- Bonding between the mother and the child is established and maintained from shortly after birth. The mother has a feeling of accomplishment and validation and the baby feels safe and secure with the skin to skin contact.

Breastfeeding mothers should pay close attention to their health and wellbeing in order to ensure that the experience is successful for both mother and infant. They should be allowed and encouraged to rest, exercise, eat adequately, avoid stressful situations, take their daily vitamins including iron, regularly visit their healthcare provider and seek early medical treatment for any illness or infection that may develop while they are breastfeeding. There are a few circumstances when breastfeeding is not recommended. These include infections in the mother such as HIV (The virus that causes AIDS), tuberculosis (Tb), typhoid fever, malaria, blood infections (septicemia), kidney infections (nephritis). Mothers who are substance abusers or suffering from post-partum psychoses should not be encouraged to breastfeed.

Although breastfeeding is one of the great wonders of motherhood, all mothers need a lot of support and encouragement from their healthcare team, family members and friends, and they should never be allowed to feel inadequate if their babies have to be supplemented with formulas at any time.

BURNS

Burn injuries are for the most part easily prevented, yet they rank second to motor vehicular accidents as the leading cause of accidental death in children. Children under the age of 4 years are at a particularly high risk of being scalded by hot water or other fluid in the home. In fact, hot tap water is one of the leading causes of burn injuries in the home, despite legislation requiring the presetting of new water heaters at 130^{oF}. It is very important that toddlers and young children are never left unattended even for a few minutes, because they will pull down kettles, pots and pans from a stove onto themselves. This type of injury can be minimized by ensuring that pots and pans are placed on the back burners and that the handles are facing the back rather than the front of the stove. Burns from electrical outlets still remain a growing concern despite the widely available inexpensive outlet covers. Children habitually put objects in their mouths and will drink anything from a bottle, therefore bleaches, kerosene and other household chemicals that can cause chemical burns to the skin, mouth, throat, lungs and other areas if swallowed, should be locked away and placed in cupboards that are out of their reach. Matches and lighters are a source of fascination to children and if given the opportunity, they will play with them. The consequences of this activity can be devastating; therefore it is of paramount importance that these objects are never left in places where they are readily available to children.

Prevention is the key but in the event of an accident there are a few first aid measures that may be taken to minimize the injury, these include:

- If a minor scald or burn occurs, then place the area under running cold tap water until the burning sensation stops. This may take 10 minutes or even more. Do not apply butter or Vaseline to the area because this will make the injury worse by trapping the heat and causing a deeper burn to the area.

- If the clothes are aflame, then the child should be placed on the ground/floor and rolled over and over until the flames go out or they may be wrapped in a rug or blanket, if readily available and rolled, to put out the flames. They should never be allowed to run, because this will cause the flames to burn even more and worsen the injury. The common saying is to "stop, drop and roll."

- Children who drink bleach or kerosene should not be induced to vomit, because this will result in the chemical burning the areas twice, as well as increasing the risk of aspiration into the lungs. Call 911 immediately and flush the mouth with water.

The degree and site of a burn injury determines the eventual outcome and long term effects on the child. Facial injuries can be disfiguring and will obviously affect the individual's perception of him or herself, resulting in a low self-esteem. Severe burns may ultimately result in the death of a child from complications such as dehydration and infection. Caution must be observed at all times when young children are at risk of being injured. Children should not be left unattended wherever candles or open flames are being used. Many families have endured the pain of losing one or more family members in the winter months because of such heating appliances.

CANKER SORES

◆

(MOUTH ULCERS)

The painful ulcers that sometimes show up in an adult's mouth can also occur in a child's mouth and when they do, they produce a lot of discomfort and feeding difficulties. They may occur anywhere inside the mouth as single or multiple sores. Initially they are red, swollen circular lesions that quickly break down to appear flattened with a reddish halo and a grayish fluid oozing from them. The common, minor ulcers range from 2–10 mm in size and usually heal without treatment within 7–10 days. However, there are some less common, major ulcers that are greater than 10 mm in size and they take 10–30 days to heal. These ulcers are sometimes confused with herpetic ulcers especially when they present in groups, but although the herpetic ulcers may be found inside the mouth, they more commonly occur on the skin near to the angle of the mouth or near to the junction of the inner and outer lips. The exact cause of these ulcers is unknown but in many instances when they recur, they tend to run in families and are associated with trauma, emotional stress, anemia, food hypersensitivity and allergies. Adolescent girls sometimes have these ulcers during the menstrual period because of the decrease in the level of progestogens, and children with crohn's or celiac disease tend to have them because of the malabsorption problems associated with those diseases. Some patients have found that sweets, nuts and chocolates precipitate canker sores.

Treatment is mainly geared towards pain relief and good oral hygiene. Although brushing the teeth may be associated with a little bleeding, it is important not to allow that to be a reason to stop, because the sores will get worse if the mouth is not kept as clean as possible. In order to prevent further injury to the gums, toothbrushes should be soft and without frays. Acetaminophen (Tylenol) and mouth rinses containing 0.2% Chlorhexidine Gluconate may be helpful in older children, while infants may benefit from the application of anesthetic gels, such as Oragel, to the affected areas prior to feeds as well as wiping the mouth with a clean, moist, soft cloth after feeding. Severe and prolonged cases usually occur in older patients and children who have underlying diseases that decrease their immunity, and they require more intense therapy with agents containing corticosteroids, colchicines, tetracycline or dapsone.

The most important things to remember are that the ulcers usually disappear after 7–10 days and the mouth must be kept as clean as possible. During the illness, the child should be encouraged to drink small amounts of fluids as often as possible in order to avoid dehydration. Avoid acidic fruit juices and fruits such as pineapple, grapes, plums, tomatoes, and citrus fruits, because they tend to cause pain when they come in contact with the ulcers. This is a "wound" that will really heal with "time."

CHICKENPOX

Chickenpox is highly contagious and is caused by a virus. Many mothers are familiar with this illness and can usually recall that their child had a mild fever and felt somewhat ill for about 1–2 days before the rash and the itching started. At first the rash appears as a few small bumps on the face, scalp or trunk but they rapidly start to look like water blisters which then dry up as scabs before they fall off and heal completely. Just when you think the rash is going away new crops will show up, but unless there are complications, they usually resolve within 1–2 weeks. The good news is that most people develop a lifelong immunity to this infection after the initial suffering. On the other hand, the virus may remain in a "resting" state in the nervous system, until something such as HIV (The virus that causes AIDS), medications such as antibiotics or even stress, causes the body's immune system to become weak, then it awakens to produce an illness commonly known as shingles.

Although there is a medication (acyclovir) that is available for the treatment of chicken pox, the American Academy of Pediatrics does not recommend its routine use in otherwise healthy children because of its questionable benefit, its relatively high cost and the low risk of complications from the illness itself. Therapy is therefore geared towards making the child feel more comfortable. This includes the use of medications to control fever (temperature above 102^{oF}) and itching. Acetaminophen (Tylenol) may be used but aspirin should be avoided due the associated complication known as Reye's syndrome, which is a disease that causes damage to the liver and the brain. Several over the counter products have been recommended to control the itching, included among these are, calamine lotion, oatmeal (Aveeno) baths, baking soda baths, and oral anti-histamines such as Benadryl. The anti-histamines have an added benefit of making the child sleep for longer periods. It is important to cut the fingernails because these children tend to scratch the lesions and if the skin becomes broken they could become infected with bacteria that could lead to complications. Keeping the skin cool will decrease the intensity of the itch; therefore keeping a wet wash cloth on hand may be very soothing. Calamine lotion cools the skin but only when it is wet, therefore it has to be applied frequently to be effective. If the calamine lotion contains an anesthetic agent such as phenol, then it should not be applied more than 3–4 times each day and should only be placed on the lesions and not the healthy skin, due to the possibility of it being absorbed through the skin. Never apply anti-itch creams or ointment that contains a steroid, because they could decrease the body's ability to fight the infection and therefore make the illness worse. Topical anti-histamines are not recommended because some children might develop an allergic reaction that will result in further complications. Daily cool showers or baths are highly recommended.

Contact your healthcare provider immediately if the lesions have yellow pus draining from them or if your child develops a high fever, cough, headache or yellow eyes (jaundice).

A chicken pox vaccine is now widely available and is routinely given to children between 12–18 months of age. Between the ages of 12 months to 12 years only one vaccine dose is required but adolescents and adults should be given 2 separate doses at least 4 weeks apart. The vaccine is not recommended for individuals who have already had chicken pox.

CIRCUMCISION

Circumcision (the removal of the penile foreskin), has been a controversial topic for as long as the practice has been around and today the ambivalence still remains. In the past the recommendation in favor of circumcision was primarily based on the premise that this would decrease the chances of developing penile cancer later in life. However, it has since been proven that if the penis is regularly cleaned in the correct manner then there is no increase in the incidence of penile cancer.

There are a few babies who are at risk of having infections of their urinary tracts because they are born with abnormalities of their kidneys and urinary system. Circumcision decreases the number of infections and is therefore recommended for these infants.

Although this is a simple surgical procedure, there are complications that may arise and parents should be informed about these before the event. The commonest problems are bleeding and infection of the site. More serious complications include narrowing of the opening of the penis, removal of insufficient or an excessive amount of the foreskin, inability to pull back the foreskin, generalized spread of infection from the circumcised site, and amputation of the tip of the penis. 0.2–3.0% of patients require a second operation.

There are certain infants who have medical reasons that dictate that they should not be circumcised. Some of these include babies whose penile opening is not at the tip but at a different part of the penis, those with a penis that is curved when erect, those with abnormalities of the foreskin and those with an extremely small penis.

There are social, cultural, religious and other reasons that may form the basis for this operation, but at this time there is no general medical recommendation that endorses the circumcision of male infants.

COMMON COLD

The common cold occurs quite frequently in childhood and is highly contagious. It is usually spread by contact with droplets or secretions from the nose and mouth. This may occur through sneezing, coughing, spitting, sharing cups and other eating utensils, hand shaking and kissing. Simple but extremely effective ways of preventing the spread of this illness include frequent hand washing, using disposable tissues for wiping nasal secretions and covering the mouth when one sneezes or coughs.

Although there are three main viruses that are associated with this illness, it may be caused by more than 200 viruses and this makes it very difficult to create a vaccine that would be of any real benefit. Children may have three to eight attacks in one year while adults may have two to four. The number of attacks usually increases when a child enters daycare or kindergarten.

The symptoms appear to be more severe in young infants because the nasal congestion prevents them from breathing and feeding properly. These infants are frequently unable to breathe through their mouths and are therefore at risk of breathing complications. It is very important to keep the nasal passages clear by using a bulb syringe to remove thick and dry secretions. When the secretions are dry, one may apply 2 drops of salt water into each nostril at a time, pausing for about 2 to 3 minutes before suctioning with the bulb syringe. This solution may be made at home by mixing one teaspoon of salt with eight ounces of water, or may be bought over the counter as saline nose drops. These drops are usually effective and are useful before meals and at bedtime. Allowing the child to lie with the head elevated will help to keep the nasal passages clear. Pillows are not to be used in young infants, therefore books or other objects may be placed beneath the head of the mattress to achieve this effect.

If the child appears to be comfortable and feeding well, then there is no need for any further treatment. However, if there is obvious discomfort due to fever, congestion, runny nose or cough, then one may treat the symptoms that are most troubling with over the counter medications. There is a vast array of these that are now available, therefore one has to read the labels to ensure that they buy the product that is specific for the symptoms that they wish to relieve.

Medications such as codeine and dextromethorphan that suppress coughing should not be used in asthmatics or in the early stages of the cold, because that is the body's way of protecting the lungs from becoming infected with the secretions that drain downward from the back of the nose. They may be useful at nights in the later stages when the cough is dry, irritative and preventing the child from sleeping. Fever reducers containing acetaminophen are recommended but aspirin should be avoided due to its association with Reye's syndrome. Decongestants help to keep the nose clear, expectorants such as guaifenesin may be helpful in the early stages when the thick mucus secretions draining at the back of the nose cause significant coughing. Lots of fluids and a cool mist humidifier may prove more useful than expectorants. Antibiotics are not indicated.

If the child appears relatively well, it may be better to treat him/her with tender loving care than with multiple medications. One should remember that some of the medications contain alcohol and that some of the side effects may be more serious than the effects of the cold itself.

CONSTIPATION IN CHILDREN

Constipation may occur at any age and the causes vary from inadequate fluid intake to structural abnormalities of the intestines. The nature and frequency of the stool must be considered when one speaks of this condition. The symptoms include straining, stools streaked with blood, small, hard pebbles, and infrequent bowel movements.

The more serious causes usually present within the first few months of life and these children should be seen and evaluated by a healthcare professional as soon as possible. The vast majority is due to dietary inadequacies and treatment may range from increasing the amount of fluid and fiber in the diet, to the use of enemas and hospitalization.

Infants who are completely breastfed may not pass stool on a daily basis, however when they do, the stool is usually very soft or even watery and abundant. This is not to be confused with constipation. This is not abnormal and may be explained by the fact that breast milk is readily absorbed and facilitates the passing of stool when necessary. These infants require no specific intervention. Infants, who are formula supplemented or totally formula fed, are more at risk of constipation, especially if they are given iron fortified formulas. A teaspoon of dark brown karo syrup added to two to three ounces of water, may prove to be a beneficial stool softener for the young infant. I do not recommend adding the syrup or any other medication to the formula, because the child may start associating the taste with the formula and this may affect his or her feeding habits.

During the period of toilet training some children, for a variety of reasons, develop the habit of withholding their stools, simply because they do not like the act or sometimes due to pain. This can result in the stools becoming even harder, larger and more difficult to pass. Chronic constipation then develops causing the walls of the rectum and lower end of the colon to become distended and less sensitive to stretch, thus decreasing the desire to pass stool and worsening the situation. When the rectum becomes overly distended, the newly formed stool from above may leak around the hard stool and result in soiling of the child's underwear. This is sometimes mistaken for diarrhea. It is important to note that the child has no control over the episodes of soiling and although it may be quite distressing, the condition is relatively easy to treat. These children may have to undergo behavior modification therapy to prevent stool retention; otherwise they may revert to their previous pattern once disimpaction has occurred.

Early recognition and intervention with preventive dietary measures can play a major role in managing this childhood problem.

CRADLE CAP/SEBORRHEIC DERMATITIS IN INFANTS

During the first few months of life, it is not uncommon to notice a patch of dry, scaly, greasy, yellow, bumpy crust, with underlying redness, on the baby's scalp. Although it may be somewhat unsightly, unless it becomes infected, it presents no threat to the baby's health and is relatively easy to treat. It is usually non-itchy and confined to the crown or mole of the head, but may occur wherever there are sebaceous glands in the body. These glands are usually located near to a hair follicle and they produce a cheesy looking secretion known as sebum.

When the scalp is affected it is usually referred to as cradle cap, in babies and dandruff in adults. Other areas of the body that may be affected include the face, neck, behind the ears, the armpits, the upper chest, the back and the groin region. If there is itching associated with the lesion, then one should suspect that the child also has another condition known as eczema or atopic dermatitis. This condition may be associated with hair loss and is sometimes confused with ringworm of the scalp, which is a fungal infection.

No one knows why cradle cap occurs in some babies but in a minority of cases it may be due to disorders of the immune system. However, these cases are usually very difficult to treat and are associated with other symptoms such as chronic diarrhea and failure to thrive.

Cradle cap may be treated with a mild baby shampoo and mineral oil or olive oil. It is usually a good idea to apply the oil to the baby's scalp at least five minutes before washing the hair. If the crust is thick, then after soaking the scalp with the oil, one may use a fine toothed comb or a toothbrush to remove the flakes prior to washing the hair. If the crusting is unusually thick, then one may allow the oil to remain on the scalp overnight before shampooing the hair. The anti-dandruff shampoos are usually quite effective in older children and adults, but are not recommended for infants under one year of age. The cases with associated itching and swelling usually respond well to the application of mild over the counter steroid ointment or lotions, which usually contain a low dose of hydro-cortisone.

If the diagnosis is correct and there are no complications, the response to treatment should be quite rapid.

CROUP

Many parents have had the frightening experience of being awakened at night by the sound of their young child being ill with a harsh and hoarse barking type of cough that ends in a strange crowing sound (stridor) as they take a breath. This phenomenon is called croup and although it presents dramatically, it is usually not as serious as it appears. A few viruses are responsible for this illness. They attack the voice box (vocal chords, larynx) and the windpipe (trachea), causing them to become swollen and inflamed. The swelling causes the air passages to become narrow and this is responsible for the hoarse cough and stridor that are the hallmarks of this disease. In a few instances the swelling might be severe enough to cause significant difficulty in breathing and these children should be treated as cases of emergency. It is more commonly seen in boys between the ages of 3–6 years and tends to occur during the colder months between fall and spring.

In the majority of cases, a few days before the cough appears, the child and sometimes another family member are noted to have mild runny nose with or without a low grade fever. The milder cases of croup can be treated at home, but if the child's condition progressively worsens then he or she should be taken to the emergency room [ER] for further evaluation and management. The red flag signs that suggest that your child needs to be taken to the ER include:

- High fever 102–104°F (39–40°C).

- Rapid worsening of the symptoms.

- Drooling, restlessness, rapid breathing or gasping for air.

- Sitting up and leaning forward.

- Pale, blue or gray appearance.

- Almost no sound when crying or talking and working hard to breathe as evidenced by flaring of the nostrils, with easy visibility of the rib cage and collar bones.

Any one of these signs could mean moderate to severe obstruction of the air passages and also that your child might have another illness such as epiglottitis or tracheitis that present in a manner that is similar to but more serious than croup. These cases should not be treated at home. It is important to note that a parent or caregiver should never attempt to look at the affected child's throat because this might worsen the condition and even result in complete closure of the airway, resulting in lack of oxygen and even death.

Managing simple cases of croup at home is easy and effective. Therapy involves exposing the child to a humidified environment. This can be achieved with the steam that results from turning on the hot water tap in a closed bathroom, or by using a vaporizer or nebulizer in the child's bedroom. Sometimes turning on the air conditioner, opening the window or taking the child outdoors for a brief period will result in improvement. Children with fever tend to breathe faster, therefore decreasing the body's temperature with a fever reducer such as acetaminophen (Tylenol), may be helpful. Dehydration should be avoided by encouraging frequent small sips of clear fluids such as Pedialyte, Gatorade, apple juice or even chicken broth. In order to prevent further obstruction of the airway from crying or talking, it is important that both the parent and the child remain as calm as possible.

Uncomplicated cases usually show improvement within minutes of exposure to humidified air and the children are almost back to normal within 2–3 days.

Having croup does not make one immune to getting another attack and in fact recurrences are relatively frequent.

DIAPER CARE

The skin of the infant is quite sensitive and easily chafed. It is therefore of paramount importance that the diaper area is kept as clean and dry as possible at all times. One needs to note that organisms thrive in moist, warm and dark areas. Therefore the diaper area is a potential breeding ground for bacteria and fungi. Diaper rash is the commonest skin disorder in infancy and it is usually most bothersome between the ages of 9–12 months. The best treatment and preventive measure for diaper rash are frequent diaper changes and cleansing of the area with a mild unscented soap, especially after a bowel movement. Other protective measures include keeping the infant's bottom naked until the rash resolves, and the use of barrier creams that provide a protective film between the skin and the feces or urine. Creams containing zinc oxide are preferred because they are soothing, adherent and promote healing. The more modern diapers provide more absorption than in the past and therefore help to prevent diaper rashes.

If your infant continues to develop diaper rash despite frequent changes, it may be a good idea to switch to cloth diapers for a brief period in order to get a true picture of how frequently he or she is passing urine. This will then provide a better guideline for the baby's caregiver, who may be underestimating the number of diaper changes that are necessary for that particular child. Regular diapers are quite absorbent, therefore the child may have passed urine several times before being noticed, resulting in the skin being wet for an extended period of time and therefore facilitating the development of a rash.

If any of the following symptoms appear it is important to seek medical help because these rashes may be due to a fungal or bacterial infection or even other skin disorders such as eczema and may therefore require more intense treatment:

- Rash persisting for more than 5 days.
- Rash associated with water boils, or bumps with pus.
- Rash associated with cracking or bleeding.
- Rash extending beyond the confines of the diaper.

Diaper wipes should be used in moderation because of the risk of a diaper rash developing from the ingredients in the wipe solution; however there are hypoallergenic ones that may cause less irritation. Dusting powders should be avoided and the plastic of the diaper should not touch the infant's skin.

DYSLEXIA

In the past and even today many children have not been able to reach their full academic potential because they have had difficulty in reading and passing examinations. They were sometimes labeled as being retarded, slow or even moronic. Today we now know and are able to recognize that some children have learning disabilities that may cause difficulties in reading and comprehension. Once they have been evaluated and diagnosed it is not unusual to overcome the specific problem with specialized training techniques.

Dyslexia is the commonest learning disability and eighty percent (80%) of children who are diagnosed as having a learning disability are dyslexic. These children have no problem understanding spoken language but they find it difficult to spell, or to read and understand a written text. When they try to read aloud they have difficulty using phonics to sound out and pronounce unfamiliar words. They spend so much time trying to figure out the correct sounds for the words, that they are unable to absorb and understand what they are reading. This difficulty is due to a lack of the ability to identify and link printed symbols to sound. This disability runs in families and appears to be due to a chromosomal abnormality. 23–65% of children who have a dyslexic parent inherit the disorder. Both boys and girls are equally affected and it does not disappear with age. Some children and adults find ways to overcome their disability on their own, but there are specific methods now available that have been developed, to assist these children at an early age. If a pre-schooler or kindergartner has difficulty playing rhyming games and learning the names for letters and numbers, then it may be a sign that the child is dyslexic and should be seen and evaluated by a child psychologist. Most of these children have average or above average intelligence and once the specific problem with phonics is identified and dealt with, their academic skills improve and they become successful in their chosen careers.

Dyslexia is not curable, but early recognition and intensive intervention are essential for improving reading skills of affected individuals. They have to be taught that words can be broken down into smaller units of sound (phonologic awareness) and that sounds (phonemes) are linked to specific letters and letter patterns (phonics). These children need a lot of practice in reading stories in order to improve their decoding skills as well as to assist them to understand what they read. Older students, such as those in college, who are diagnosed later in life, also need professional assistance and they should be allowed extra time for reading and writing assignments and examinations. This is because they may improve their reading accuracy but not their speed. They may find it easier to cope if they have access to lecture notes and tutorials, and are allowed to use tape recorders in the classroom, audio taped books and laptop computers with spell checkers. Best results are obtained from examinations if they are allowed to sit in a separate quiet room and are given essays or other alternatives to multiple choice questions.

EARACHES AND EAR INFECTION IN CHILDREN

Pain in the ear is one of the commonest complaints in childhood and is usually a sign of inflammation in either the outer or middle parts of the ear. However, it is important to note that not every child who rubs or pulls the ear has an ear infection; there are times when the problem may originate from the teeth, the back of the throat or other areas on the face. An earache that is associated with fever may suggest the presence of an ear infection, but this can only be confirmed by a healthcare professional after adequate evaluation of the child. Pus draining from the ear, redness and swelling of the canal or outer portions of the ear, or the presence of a foreign body inserted in the ear canal are signs that make the diagnosis quite obvious. Sometimes an earache may be associated with other signs and symptoms that suggest the presence of a complication or a more serious underlying problem. Included among these are: clear liquid draining from the ear, hearing loss, ringing in the ear (tinnitus), dizziness (vertigo), facial weakness or paralysis and abnormal movements of the eyes (nystagmus). A pediatrician or an ear nose and throat surgeon (an otolaryngologist) should see any child with these problems.

Middle ear infections are ranked as the commonest childhood infection in the United States and may occur at any age. They are more commonly seen in situations where children are at a higher risk of getting an upper respiratory tract infection, such as the common cold. This includes during the winter months, between the ages of 6 and 13 months, children who attend day-care nurseries, children who are exposed to second-hand smoke, non breast-fed children and those children whose siblings or parents also had ear infections. Young children are also at a higher risk because their Eustachian tube which is relatively short, wide and straight versus the adult tube that is long, narrow and curved, tends to get swollen and blocked when a child has a cold, sinusitis or even an allergy attack. This tube connects the middle ear to the back of the throat and is responsible for normalizing the pressure, by draining fluid from and allowing air to flow into and out of the middle ear. A swollen Eustachian tube cannot function properly, and this increases the chances of a child developing a middle ear infection. Most children outgrow their tendency to have ear infections, but there are a few that continue to have this problem even into adulthood.

Viruses or bacteria may be responsible for an ear infection, therefore your healthcare professional needs to evaluate the child and make a determination concerning the need for antibiotics. Some children who tend to have frequent or persistent ear infections may benefit from having tubes inserted into the ear-drums as well as by taking antibiotics for a prolonged period, sometimes as long as three months.

Although there are a wide variety of complications that may occur, the most feared are meningitis and deafness. It is of paramount importance that children take their medications as prescribed by their health care provider and return for their follow-up visits until they are given a clean bill of health.

FEEDING SCHEDULE FOR AN INFANT

Among the many advantages of breast-feeding, the main ones include mother-infant bonding and the transmission of infection fighting materials called antibodies. The newborn infant is better served by feeding him or her breast milk for the first six months of life. However this is not always practical for the mother and or the infant. In these cases the mother needs to know that there are various nutritionally complete formulas that are specially designed for infants at different ages and stages of their life.

There are many recommended feeding schedules, but based on the infant's physiological, anatomical and neurological development (age and stage), my preferred recommendation is as follows:

0–4 months: Breast milk and or formula plus water, when necessary.

4–6 months: Introduction of a single grain cereal such as rice.

6–7 months: Introduction of a fruit, such as a freshly crushed banana and fruit juice such as freshly squeezed and strained orange juice.

7–8 months: Introduction of a single-ingredient vegetable such as carrot.

9–10 months: Introduction of meat such as chicken.

After 12 months: Introduction of fresh whole milk.

Note Carefully: The general rule when introducing new foods is to offer one new single-ingredient food at a time and to stick to this new food daily for at least 3–5 days, in order to detect and identify any allergen or food sensitivity. Different foods should be added in a gradual manner and withdrawn if a negative reaction develops. Do not add sugar or any other sweetener to the baby's formula.

When new foods are introduced at an inappropriately early age, the body's digestive and immune systems are not equipped to handle them and the body may react in a negative manner. Some parents think that their child should be introduced to solids as early as possible to facilitate sleeping through the night, but this has not been proven scientifically and may even result in feeding difficulties, childhood obesity and the development of food allergies.

It is a good idea to offer the baby some water after feeding when they are too young to have their teeth brushed. Never let a child go to sleep with a bottle of milk or juice in his or her mouth, because this may result in problems ranging from "bottle teeth caries" to aspiration into the lungs, which could be a life threatening situation. Time and patience are two key ingredients to feeding a baby correctly and these will prove to be of long term benefit to everyone.

FETAL ALCOHOL SYNDROME

✦

(FAS)

The fetal alcohol syndrome (FAS) is a classic example of the unfairness of life, in that the child suffers because of the mother's abuse of alcohol during pregnancy. This disorder is totally preventable, yet it affects 1–2 of every 1000 children that are born alive in the United States of America. It also accounts for 10–20 % of the cases of mental retardation and about 17 % of the cases of cerebral palsy.

There are several features that may be present in a child whose mother drinks alcohol during her pregnancy and the degree and number of problems vary with the quantity of alcohol that she drinks each day. Mothers who drink more than 56–84 g of absolute alcohol (approximately 4–6 beers, 4–6 glasses of wine, or 4–6 mixed drinks) per day are considered to be heavy drinkers, and their babies are most often and more severely affected. When all the features of the syndrome are present, the child is said to have FAS, however, if the mother were a moderate drinker, the child may only have a few of the abnormalities, and they would be described as having fetal alcohol effects (FAE). In fact, 30% of the infants whose mothers are heavy drinkers will have FAS and 50–70% will have FAE, while 14% of infants of moderate drinkers have abnormalities at birth. It is important to note that women who do not drink may also have children with birth defects, but this only occurs in about 9% of newborns.

The FAS is responsible for significant growth retardation, before and after birth; both the head and body are smaller than expected. There are several facial abnormalities which include:

: Shortening of the distance between the eyebrows
: Folds of skin that extend on either side of the nose bridge from the eyebrow or eyelid area to cover the inner part of the opening of the eye, (epicanthic folds)
: Under-developed cheekbones

: Small chin, a thin upper lip, long flat mid-face, long flat area between the nose and the upper lip (philtrum), abnormal growth of facial hair and weakness of the upper eyelids, resulting in difficulty in opening the eyes to their widest capacity (ptosis).

Other problems involve different systems of the body such as heart abnormalities; commonly a "hole" in the heart (a communication between the right and left chambers), abnormalities of the joints and limbs, resulting in some degree of restriction of movement, delayed developmental milestones, and mental retardation of varying degrees.

There are other abnormalities that are also associated with alcohol abuse during pregnancy and because the full syndrome is not present, it is sometimes difficult to diagnose FAE if the mother denies drinking alcohol.

There is no treatment that will reverse the effects of the alcohol in these children but their lives can be made more comfortable by early intervention and assistance where necessary. Speech, physical and occupational therapy, as well as behavior modification and special education programs should be recommended. Children with FAS should have frequent hearing tests and dental checks as well as preventive healthcare visits and their parents or caregivers should receive psychological support and counseling.

There is no absolutely safe level for the amount of alcohol that a pregnant woman may drink before the infant is at risk of developing an abnormality. There is also no way of knowing which infant will or will not be affected, therefore the best advice is not to drink alcohol during pregnancy.

FEVER

When the body is in the process of fighting an infection it produces heat which is called a fever. This heat helps to kill the viruses or bacteria that are invading the body. When a child has a fever it is more important to find out what is causing it rather than trying to reduce it. In most instances the infection is usually not serious but there are a few cases where it may be due to a potentially life-threatening illness. The degree of the fever is not a true indicator of the seriousness of the condition; therefore it is always better to seek medical advice whenever a child has a fever. It is safe to assume that an ill-looking child who also has a fever might need more urgent attention than one who is alert, active and feeding well.

A high fever can occasionally cause the child to have a seizure. This is usually a frightening experience but it only lasts for a very short time, and it will not cause brain damage. It tends to occur in families and may happen again when the child gets another illness that is associated with a fever. The important thing to remember is to stay calm, do not leave the child, allow the child to lie on a flat surface such as the ground and keep the airway open by positioning the head to the side and holding it in an upward and backward position, (hyper-extension). Never try to put an object such as a finger or spoon into the mouth of a child who is having a seizure, and do not try to stop it by restraining the child's body. A physician should see any child, who has had a seizure, especially on the first occasion. These children should be given fever reducers at an earlier stage than others, in an attempt to prevent the recurrence of a seizure.

In most cases it is not always necessary to reduce the fever. However if it is very high, example above 104 ^{o}F/40 ^{o}C, then the child might feel quite uncomfortable and weak. In such a situation it would be helpful to give a fever reducer such as acetaminophen, which is found in Tylenol and other over the counter preparations. Aspirin should be avoided because of its association with the development of Reye's syndrome when given to some children who were incubating the chickenpox and other viruses that were associated with a fever. Reye's syndrome causes liver and brain failure and could result in death. In my opinion one should not give a child aspirin unless a healthcare provider prescribes it for a specific illness such as Rheumatic Fever.

<u>Note Carefully</u>: A child who has a fever within the first 28 days of life should be treated as a case of emergency, and do not observe a child with a fever for longer than 48 hours without seeking the advice of a healthcare provider.

FIFTH DISEASE

Fifth disease received its name simply because it was the fifth class of childhood infections that was associated with a rash. It is commoner during the winter and spring months and is caused by a virus that is spread via secretions from the mouth and nose. An infected child does not appear very ill, but may have a few symptoms before the appearance of the rash. These include mild fever, headache, and symptoms of the common cold. In the early stage, the child's face appears flushed, resulting in the typical "slapped cheek" appearance, which makes it easier to diagnose. However as time progresses, the rash rapidly spreads to involve the trunk and upper parts of the arms and legs. The appearance then changes from being evenly red to some clearing in the central areas giving rise to a rather lacy pattern. The palms and soles are not usually affected and there may or may not be mild itching and some swelling of the lymph glands. The rash may appear and disappear over a period of 1–3 weeks and may be worsened by stress, exercise, heat and exposure to sunlight. The commonest complications are joint pains and arthritis and these mainly affect older adolescents and adults.

There is neither an anti-viral medication nor any vaccine for fifth's disease but the illness usually gets better without side effects. There is no need to prevent a child with this disease from attending school because by the time the rash appears and the diagnosis is made, he/she has already passed the infectious stage. Pregnant women who are in contact with an infected child are at risk of developing complications and should be evaluated by their obstetrician.

FROSTBITE

Playing outdoors is a healthy way for kids to exercise and have fun; however, during the colder months they are at risk of being over exposed to the low temperatures which could result in cold injury to different parts of their bodies. The areas that are most commonly affected are the ears, nose, cheeks, fingers and toes. Initially there will be warning signs that the body's ability to maintain a normal temperature is failing and if these are ignored, then the child may develop a frostbite injury. Some of the warning signs include redness, followed by tingling or stinging, then pain. If the child ignores these feelings and remains outdoors, then there may be progression to a full-blown case of frostbite. The cold air causes actual freezing of the blood cells of the affected areas and the injury may range from mild to severe. The affected area appears cold, numb, white and hard. If immediate relief is not available, in extreme cases, the child could actually lose a limb.

When treating an individual with frostbite it is very important to remember that one should never rub the area and definitely not rub it with ice or snow, because rubbing will cause the ice crystals beneath the skin, to damage the skin cells. If the injury occurs at home, an excellent way to re-warm the body is by placing the child in a bathtub that is filled with warmed water (40–42^{oC} or 104–108^{oF}). If the fingers and toes are affected, then they should be kept in the water until the child regains full feeling in them. This might take 15–20 minutes or even longer at times. It is important that the temperature of the water is determined to be safe by an adult and not the affected child whose body parts are numb and unable to feel pain, because the child might burn himself/herself with very hot water without even realizing it. Once full feeling has returned, the child should be seen and evaluated by a healthcare professional, who will determine the need for further management.

If the injury occurs in a situation where the above therapy is not possible, remove the wet clothes and replace them with dry ones, then commence re-warming by placing the affected area/s against unaffected areas of the body while the child is on the way to the nearest healthcare facility. If there is a possibility that the area will refreeze after thawing, it is better not to allow it to thaw in the first place, because re-freezing will increase the chances of permanent damage to the tissues than would a single freezing episode.

If the skin becomes swollen and painful, the child may be given some medication containing acetaminophen (Tylenol) or ibuprofen (Advil, Motrin). Once re-warming has occurred it is important to keep the area dry and clean to prevent infection. If the skin is broken do not cover the affected area because oxygen from the air will aid in the healing process. There should not be any type of pressure or contact to the area and the child should be placed on bed rest until the swelling subsides. Close attention should be paid to the child's nutritional status and once recovery has commenced, physical therapy should be started in order to restore normal range of motion. It is not unusual to regain complete recovery even with severe injuries.

Children should always be supervised and when they are playing in the cold outdoors, an adult should monitor them and summon them indoors periodically for warming. Instead of just a shirt and a heavy coat they should be properly dressed with a hat and scarf or a neck gaiter, water resistant gloves or mittens, wool or polypropylene socks, snow boots with removable liners that can be dried out, layered clothing which includes long thermal underwear topped by a turtle neck, a sweater and a water resistant jacket. Children should play in groups of two or more and each child should be assigned a buddy who is responsible for looking at the other child's ears, nose and cheeks for color changes such as redness, paleness or blueness. As with any injury, prevention is the key.

GASTRO-ENTERITIS

❖

(VOMITING & DIARRHEA)

Gastro-enteritis is a common occurrence among toddlers and pre-schoolers. There are many causes but in most cases it is due to a viral infection. The illness tends to spread very quickly because these children do not pay close attention to personal hygiene, such as washing their hands before eating and after using the toilet. They also tend to share objects that are placed in the mouth and they may even put their hands in their diapers or underpants and then put their fingers in their mouths. Their adult care-givers may also be guilty of not adequately washing their hands between diaper changes and before preparing meals.

There is no cure for this illness but there are ways of preventing and controlling the spread of it to others as well as preventing death due to dehydration. The principal method of controlling its spread is by hand washing and a major deterrent to its onset is the anti-viral (rotavirus) vaccine that protects infants who are at a higher risk of developing complications from gastro-enteritis.

The most important part of the treatment is to ensure that the patient is given the correct type of fluids in frequent, small amounts to prevent dehydration and that the re-introduction of solids is appropriate both in terms of type of food and its timing.

Initially, the child should be given an oral rehydration solution that replaces the water and salts that are lost in the vomitus and the stools. The World Health Organization (WHO) and the United Nations Children's Fund (UNICEF) have recommended the use of a widely available solution that can be bought over the counter. They are marketed under different trade names, such as Pedialyte and Rehydralyte. The fluid should be given in small amounts, preferably by spoon and in some cases as frequently as every 10–15 minutes. Ideally this should be done under the guidance of a healthcare provider. It requires time and patience on the part of the parent or caregiver, but its advantages far outweigh the disadvantages of hospitalization.

Apart from the rehydration fluid, other foods should be withheld for the first 24 hours, and then the next day the child should be offered fluids or bland solids that are age appropriate. A young infant may be given breast milk or diluted formula while an older child may be given rice cereal, potatoes, or bananas.

Anti-diarrheal agents such as Kaopectate and Lomotil should not be given to these children and in some cases they may prove to be very dangerous. Antibiotics are of no value in the treatment of these viral illnesses.

There are a few instances when the illness is caused by bacteria and in such cases antibiotics would be beneficial, however these cases should be diagnosed and cared for directly by a competent healthcare provider.

GROWTH PATTERNS

Growth is not a static process and there is a wide range of normal variation. Changes in body proportions depend on physique as well as rates of growth of different body parts.

It is important to note that the brain attains adult size at a much earlier age than the face or the rest of the body, therefore the head may appear relatively large in a young child. The extremities also grow at a faster rate than the trunk. Normally the sitting height reflects approximately 70% of body length in the newborn infant, 57% at 3 years, and about 50% at the time of the first period in a girl and at about 15 years in boys. Following this period there is then a mild increase of 1–2–percentage points, as the trunk continues to grow after the extremities have finished growing. There are reference standards available for weights and heights for children of given ages and stages of development and they show a wide variation of normal values. The best index of general growth is an individual's bone age as determined from x-rays.

Needless to say, genetic, ethnic, and environmental or socioeconomic factors also play significant roles in the growth potential of a child. A child who does not receive adequate nutrition is at risk of not attaining his or her growth potential and a child who is overfed is at risk of obesity and its negative health associations.

HAND, FOOT AND MOUTH DISEASE

Although other areas may also be involved, as the name suggests, this disease mainly affects the hands, feet and mouth. It is more commonly seen in the summer and fall months and more often affects younger children than older ones. It is caused by a virus that gets into the body through the mouth and travels to the intestines and the respiratory tract, where it grows and multiplies before entering the blood stream, which takes it to different areas of the body.

The disease symptoms vary, depending on where the virus eventually lodges. Ulcers measuring about 4–8 mm in size usually develop on the tongue and the inner lining of the mouth. The lesions on the hands and feet measure 3–7 mm are usually tender and look like water blisters. Quite often the buttocks are also affected and the lesions usually appear as reddish bumps. There is no specific treatment for this illness, but the lesions usually disappear after about 7–10 days.

Having one attack does not produce immunity and some children have been known to get repeated attacks. It is important to prevent the child from scratching the affected areas, because if the skin becomes broken, a secondary bacterial infection could occur and this may eventually cause damage to the kidneys or other organs.

This disease may sometimes be complicated by other severe illnesses such as viral meningitis, encephalitis and even paralysis. As with most viral diseases, the key to prevention is frequent hand washing and proper disposal of diapers by caregivers. Children should be encouraged to wash their hands after using the toilet and before eating.

HEAD LICE

Head lice remain a major public health hazard and are relatively common in pre-schoolers, elementary aged children and older individuals with long unkempt hair. It is readily spread by close contact with infected individuals, their clothing, bed linens, combs, brushes, and even furniture. It is usually associated with conditions of overcrowding and less than adequate personal hygiene.

The adult lice may not be easy to see but if the head is thoroughly searched one may see them on the scalp. The eggs or nits are more easily visible on the shaft of the hair, about an inch away from the scalp. They are most commonly located above the ears and at the back of the head above the neck. This condition is accompanied by severe itching and the scratching may result in a secondary skin infection with associated swelling of the lymph glands. There may also be a skin rash on the neck and ears.

Treatment involves vigorous shampooing of the scalp and adjacent areas with a 1–% gamma benzene hexachloride shampoo, such as kwell, for 4–5 minutes followed by thorough rinsing. Any remaining nits may be removed with a fine-toothed comb. If this proves to be difficult then rinsing the hair with a 1:1 solution of vinegar and water, and then repeating the combing procedure may loosen them. It may be necessary to repeat the treatment in 1 week because some nits may survive the initial application. There are over the counter applications, such as nix, that do not require re-treatment. However, their safety has not been established in pregnant and nursing mothers as well as infants less than two years of age.

Whenever possible, brushes and combs should be discarded, or otherwise thoroughly washed in hot, boiling water. Bed linens and clothing should be dry-cleaned or laundered in very hot water.

HENOCH-SCHONLEIN PURPURA

✦

(HSP)

Henoch-schonlein purpura is a relatively common disease that affects small blood vessels and usually follows an upper respiratory tract infection, such as a cold. It is commoner in the winter months and boys between the ages of 2–8 years of age are affected twice as often as girls. The exact cause of this disease is not known but it appears to be linked with the immune system.

The child may present with signs and symptoms that appear suddenly or slowly over a period of weeks or even months. The typical presentation is the appearance of a rash that begins as pinkish, raised and flattened lesions that initially loose their color for a short while (blanch), when pressure is applied to them, then later progress to appear as purplish blotches that look like bruises, before changing to a rusty brown color prior to their disappearance. They occur in crops and usually last between 3–10 days, but they may appear at intervals between 3–4 months. In rare cases the rash may continue to reappear over a period of years. There may be swelling of the area before the rash appears and the commonest parts of the body that are affected include below the waist, over the buttocks, the eyelids, lips, scrotum, the back of the hands and feet, and the back of the scalp and trunk in babies. Most children will have involvement of their kidneys, intestines and joints and these may manifest themselves in varying ways. When the joints are affected there is arthritis mainly involving the knees and ankles. They usually heal after a few days and there is no permanent damage or deformity, but the problem may reappear at a later date. Intestinal involvement may mimic acute appendicitis and quite a few patients have undergone surgery because of the symptoms. The child usually complains of intermittent, abdominal cramps as well as diarrhea that may or may not be associated with blood in the stools. In some cases there may even be vomiting of bright red blood. On several occasions there may be a complication known as intussusception, which is a condition where the gut becomes obstructed because the lower portion slides into the upper portion right next to it and therefore prevents flow of blood, fluid and food from getting through the affected area. The child with this condition usually has a slimy, bloody stool that looks like currant jelly, shortly after a bout of abdominal pain. This may be treated by a special x-ray using a white liquid known as barium (barium enema) or by immediate surgery.

Involvement of the kidney may result in decreased urine output, headaches, swelling of the eyelids and other symptoms that are indicative of damaged kidneys. Any system or organ of the body may become involved and there are children who sometimes present with enlarged liver, spleen and lymph glands. The more severe cases may affect the brain and this could result in seizures, weakness of certain body parts and even coma and death.

Treatment is based on providing relief from the symptoms until the body heals itself. When diarrhea is present, it is important that the child gets adequate and appropriate fluids, such as Pedialyte, to prevent dehydration and the diet should be simple such as jell-o, broth, or dry toast and not contain any seasoning, spices or grease. Acetaminophen (Tylenol) or ibuprofen (Motrin, Advil) will provide satisfactory relief from swelling, pain and fever. Rest and elevation of the areas involved with the swelling will help to decrease the amount and duration of the accumulation of the fluid. Your child's doctor may prescribe some steroid containing medication that usually brings dramatic relief of symptoms, especially when the brain and intestines are involved.

Although this disease may affect many organs and can cause significant illness, most children recover completely and only on rare occasions complications of the kidneys, intestines and brain result in prolonged illness or death. It is of paramount importance that children be seen and evaluated by a health care provider at the onset of symptoms of HSP.

HICCUPS

Almost every baby has suffered from the hiccups at some stage of infancy and although it is annoying, it is usually not life threatening. There are different triggers for hiccups but the underlying cause is any form of irritation that results in a rhythmic contraction of the diaphragm muscle that separates the chest from the abdomen.

The commonest irritant in babies is related to feeding problems such as swallowing too fast, swallowing excess air, indigestion or reflux of food from the stomach up through the esophagus. In the older child, laughing when the stomach is empty, excessive tiredness, and drinking or eating too fast may trigger hiccups. In a few cases prolonged hiccups may be due to serious underlying diseases that could actually affect the life of the child. Included among these are: apnea (periods of no breathing activity), tumors, injuries or infections of the brain, pneumonia and other infections of the lung and heart, intoxication with alcohol and other drugs. Unusual triggers such as over-breathing or a foreign body in the ear canal may also cause hiccups.

There is really no scientifically proven cure for the common hiccups, but there are certain maneuvers that have shown relatively consistent results. These include:

- Encouraging the baby to burp up excess air by holding him or her in an upright position against your shoulder whilst gently patting his or her back.

- Encouraging the older child to hold his/her breath for the count of ten.

- Allowing the child to swallow water or other liquid without taking a breath for the period that would correspond to having 2 or 3 hiccups.

- Distracting the child for a few minutes.

- Ensuring that when feeding an infant, the size of the hole in the nipple is neither too small nor too large. The nipple hole is adequate if the formula drips out when the bottle is turned upside down, rather than flows freely or allows no dripping at all.

- A spoonful of sugar may or may not stop the hiccups but will definitely make an older child feel better, and bear in mind that if everything fails, the hiccups will eventually disappear on their own.

IMMUNIZATION SCHEDULE

Immunization is the single most effective measure used to prevent infections and has played a very significant part in improving the quality and length of life of people all over the globe. The immunization schedule that is used internationally is recommended by the committee on infectious diseases of the American Academy of Pediatrics and the immunization practices advisory committee of the United States public health service. Although there might be a few exceptions and contraindications in specific circumstances, the following schedule is applicable to infants and children worldwide. There are updated variations to this schedule, but the basic guide for the recommended age ranges and time intervals when the vaccines should be administered is outlined below.

AGE	IMMUNIZATIONS
BIRTH	HBV
2 MONTHS	DTP HIB *OPV/IPV HBV
4 MONTHS	DTP HIB *OPV/IPV
6 MONTHS	DTP HIB HBV
12–15 MONTHS	MMR VAR HIB
15–18 MONTHS	DTP *OPV/IPV
18 MONTHS	any vaccines missed between birth and 15 months should be made up at this visit.
4 TO 6 YEARS	DTP *OPV/IPV MMR VAR[1]
11 TO 12 YEARS	HBV[2] TD MMR[3] VAR[1]
13 TO 16 YEARS	HBV[2] TD MMR[3] VAR[4]

*OPV should not be given to immunocompromised individuals because, being live, it is possible that the polio virus may revert to the wild form and therefore place these individuals at risk of contracting the disease itself.

DTP: DIPHTHERIA, TETANUS, PERTUSSIS (Whooping cough)
HBV: HEPATITIS B VACCINE
HIB: HAEMOPHILUS INFLUENZAE TYPE B
MMR: MEASLES, MUMPS, RUBELLA
OPV: ORAL POLIO VIRUS VACCINE—[live attenuated]
IPV: INACTIVATED/KILLED POLIO VIRUS VACCINE
TD: TETANUS DIPHTHERIA BOOSTER
VAR: VARICELLA (Chickenpox)

[1]GIVE ONE DOSE VARICELLA IF NOT ALREADY IMMUNIZED.
[2]BEGIN HEPATITIS B VACCINE SERIES IF NOT GIVEN IN CHILD-HOOD.
[3]GIVE MMR TWO-DOSE SERIES IF NOT ALREADY IMMUNIZED.
[4]GIVE VARICELLA TWO-DOSE SERIES IF NOT ALREADY IMMU-NIZED.

INFANTILE COLIC

This term conjures up the picture of a young infant crying and assuming the posture of someone who is experiencing severe, cramping abdominal pain. The child is usually between the ages of 3 days and 3 months and does not have a fever, rash, vomiting, diarrhea or any other symptom that suggests a source of infection. The abdomen is sometimes distended and there may be some relief when the baby passes gas. The cause is basically unknown and therefore there is no cure. The reassuring fact is that the problem is short-lived and it disappears almost as suddenly and dramatically as it appears. It usually lasts no longer than the first three months of life and it is not life threatening.

Many theories have been forwarded for its cause and different treatment modalities have been offered. However, there is nothing that works consistently for all children. Gripe water has not been shown to have any curative value and it is important to read the label, because some of the brands contain alcohol, which is not recommended for this age group. Some parents report temporary relief with simethicone drops, which apparently help to break up gas pockets in the gut. Milk allergy has been theorized, but unless there is proof or strong evidence to suggest that the child is allergic to cow's milk-based formulas, there is really no need to switch to a soy formula. The natural urge to feed a crying child should be resisted because overfeeding will lead to over distension of the stomach, resulting in further discomfort, which will be an added reason for crying.

In many instances, avoiding situations that produce anxiety or parental conflicts have proven to be beneficial. Soothing movements such as rocking, walking or taking a ride in the car have had some degree of success. This has been the source of anecdotes by pediatricians who have been called out by an anxious parent in the middle of the night only to have the child calm down and go to sleep enroute to the hospital.

One of the problems associated with colic is that after its disappearance, some parents continue to respond to every type of crying sound that the infant makes. This can result in the development of sleeping difficulties and excessive crying in order to seek attention. After 3–4 months, parents need to learn how to differentiate between a cry that indicates the need to sleep, play or have some discomfort relieved. At this age infants should be allowed to find ways to soothe themselves to sleep in order to establish a healthy sleep pattern. Over stimulation by parents may be so enjoyable that the child fights sleep until it gets to the point where fussiness develops from being overly tired. He or she then has to be actively soothed to sleep. Infants should be given less attention at sleep time and this might mean ignoring them when they cry due to tiredness. Allowing the child to find ways to sleep unassisted may be difficult in the early stages but after a few weeks the crying will disappear and the baby will be less fussy and more content.

INFECTIOUS MONONUCLEOSIS

◆

(KISSING DISEASE, GLANDULAR FEVER)

Most of us are familiar with the term "Kissing disease." This serves as a reminder that the virus that causes infectious mononucleosis may be spread through saliva. In fact, it is usually spread by close contact with secretions from the mouth or genital tract of an infected person. In a child-care setting, the constant placing of objects in the mouth makes it very easy for the virus to spread from one child to the next. Although the virus that causes infectious mononucleosis may be present in over 95% of the people in the world, the typical symptoms do not usually occur in children younger than 4 years and adults older than 40 years of age. It is most commonly seen in older children, adolescents and young adults.

It is also known as glandular fever because it not only causes fever and fatigue, but also swelling of most of the lymph glands of the body. This includes the tonsils (sore throat), liver (enlarged liver) and spleen (enlarged spleen). The typical picture is that of a young adult who complains of a sore throat, fever, headache, weakness, tiredness, nausea, abdominal pain, muscle aches and a general feeling of being ill. This may last for 1–2 weeks then the sore throat and fever may get worse. Most patients seek medical advice at this stage because they feel so very ill. Unfortunately, there is no cure, but the use of medications such as acetaminophen (Tylenol) or ibuprofen (Advil) for pain and fever may relieve the symptoms. Gargling with salt water gives temporary relief to the sore throat and adequate fluids will prevent dehydration. Bed rest is recommended for those cases that have severe fatigue. Ampicillin or Amoxicillin should not be given because they may cause a rash to appear all over the patient's body. Complications may occur in some cases resulting in spontaneous bleeding, anemia, seizures and meningitis, a short course of steroids such as prednisone, may provide relief. Anti-viral medication may be given to decrease the number of viruses in the individual, but it does not reduce the severity or duration of the symptoms nor alter the eventual outcome of the patient.

The good news is that the individual usually gets better after about 2–4 weeks and although for a few weeks to about six months, there may be spells of fatigue and a feeling of being unwell, the full blown picture does not reappear.

LYME DISEASE

Lyme disease is one of the potential hazards of enjoying the great outdoors. It commonly occurs during the summer and is caused by an organism known as Borrelia that is transmitted to humans through the bite of an infected deer tick.

Children between the ages of 5–10 years appear to be more susceptible to this disease than are older children and adults. This may partly be due to the fact that older individuals will feel the bite and remove the tick before it transmits the Borrelia into the skin. The tick has to feed for a long time, between 36–72 hours, before the organism is transmitted into the skin of a person who has been bitten.

An infected child may or may not have any symptoms for up to a month after the bite, therefore the diagnosis may be difficult because no-one may have remembered or even associated the bite with the illness. The disease may present in different ways and may occur in early or late stages. The earliest sign is a rash that begins at the site of the bite, but which later spreads in a circular form and may even be mistaken for ringworm. It may or may not be itchy or painful and may occur anywhere on the body but it is most commonly found in the armpits, around the navel, in the groin and on the thigh.

Treatment is simple and effective, but due to misdiagnoses and delayed diagnoses there is a general feeling that this disease is difficult to treat. Effective antibiotics include Doxycycline, Amoxicillin, Erythromycin or Cefuroxime.

The importance of prevention cannot be overstressed. If one cannot wear clothing that will cover the extremities of the body, then it is important to be vigilant about checking the body for any tick that may have attached itself for a feed and removing it before it is able to transmit the infection. Ticks should be forcibly removed rather that being slapped onto the surface of the skin.

MIGRAINE HEADACHES

Migraine headaches tend to run in families and before ten years of age, boys are more often affected than girls. However, after this age it is the girls who present more commonly with this problem.

The cause of migraine still remains a mystery, but there is evidence that there are high levels of certain substances such as serotonin, that act on the blood vessels surrounding the brain, causing them to contract and relax intermittently, resulting in the throbbing pain that is so typical of migraine. There are certain personality traits and associated features that make one person more likely to be affected than another. Included among these are: a family history of migraine or problems affecting certain blood vessels in the body, food allergies, stress, and individuals with high achievement personality traits.

The different manifestations of migraine make it sometimes difficult to recognize and diagnose. They include common and classic migraine, migraine variants, cluster headaches, and complicated migraine. Most children present with the common form of migraine which is usually a throbbing or pounding type of headache that affects the front or side of the head and may last for 1 to over 24 hours. Quite commonly there is nausea, vomiting, abdominal pain and even fever associated with it and less frequently there may be other symptoms such as light-headedness, pallor, fear or avoidance of light, noise and certain odors as well as a sensation of pins and needles in the hands and feet.

Those children who present with the classic form of migraine usually experience a sensation, known as an aura, before the actual headache. There may be visual or other sensory perceptions which include blurred vision, flashing lights, brilliant white zigzag lines, irregular distortion of objects or even a sensation of a distorted body image, vertigo, a feeling of pins and needles around the mouth and numbness of the hands and feet. The common type of headache usually follows the aura. A few children may present with no headache but instead they may have recurrent episodes of any of the following symptoms: vomiting, confusion, hyperactivity, disorientation, unresponsiveness, memory disturbances and lethargy. Interestingly, the symptoms tend to have a sort of cyclical pattern and may last from hours to days but tend to disappear after a deep sleep. In these cases it may be very difficult to arrive at a diagnosis without a positive family history of migraine headaches.

Cluster headaches and the complicated migraine are uncommon in children.

Complicated migraine is associated with weakness or paralysis of certain parts of the body during and after the headache and may be confused with the symptoms of a brain tumor, drug abuse, toxins or a stroke.

All cases of migraine have features that appear to be uniformly similar. These include: cycles that coincide with the menstrual period in adolescent girls (around the time of ovulation or around the time of the blood flow), following periods of intense exercise, following a stressful experience such as school examinations, precipitated by certain foods or odors and relieved by sleep. In some cases affected children will know that a migraine will be coming on because they experience cravings for certain foods, excessive sleepiness, mood swings or irritability.

The management of migraine involves avoiding situations or substances that trigger an attack and giving painkillers such as acetaminophen (Tylenol) or ibuprofen (Motrin), for the acute attacks. If vomiting is a manifestation, then an anti-vomiting medication such as Dimenhydrinate (Dramamine) may be necessary. Older children who have classic migraine may be given ergotamine preparations to ward off an attack as soon as the aura symptoms appear. Those children who are unable to attend school and have more than 2 to 4 severe attacks per month may benefit from preventive medication on a continuous daily basis, during the school year. Several medications are used in adults but in children the beta-blocker, known as Propranolol is the most popular.

There are several pediatric headache clinics that are now employing social workers who receive special training in pain management and they work with affected children who have been shown to respond quite positively to behavior therapy involving self-relaxation and biofeedback techniques. In many cases this results in a decreased need for medication. The good news is that after the age of 10 years, more than half of the children tend to outgrow their migraine attacks.

NEAR-DROWNING/ DROWNING

Water is one of the most life giving and at the same time, one of the most deadly elements in nature. The summer months are renowned for the number of people who either drown or nearly drown while swimming, diving or simply being in a body of water. Below the age of 4 years, children are at an increased risk of drowning or becoming submerged in water, therefore it is extremely important that supervising adults remain alert and aware of the children in their care at all times. Even small buckets pose a threat for small toddlers, because they may fall headlong into a bucket and then find it difficult to free themselves. Bathtubs and swimming pools are also famous for being the sites of many drowning and near-drowning accidents in the home. Boys tend to be more daring and eager to explore their surroundings; hence it is not surprising to note that they also tend to be affected more than girls.

Near-drowning is the term that describes a situation in which an individual survives for at least 24 hours after an accidental submersion. Unfortunately, about 50% of these survivors suffer some form of severe damage to their brain and nervous system, because it is much easier to revive a child's heart than the brain. Whenever a child is found submerged in a body of water, it is imperative that emergency resuscitative measures be started immediately, even before the child is taken out of the water. The first and most important step is to ensure that there is nothing blocking the airway (breathing passage) and then starting mouth to mouth breathing. Depending on the situation, there may be the possibility of injury to the spine; therefore the rescuer has to try to keep the head and spine as straight as possible to avoid damage to the spinal cord. As soon as the child is removed from the water, the rescuer should listen for a heartbeat and check for a pulse. If there is no heartbeat or pulse, then efforts at heart compression should be started along with the on-going mouth to mouth breathing and help should be sought for further assistance. Another person, if available, should call 911, but if there is no one else around, then the rescuer may have to stop for a very brief period to make the call. It is important not to panic and to continue resuscitative efforts until the ambulance team takes over. Do not try to squeeze the water out of the chest by using the Heimlich maneuver or some other approach, because this could cause the child to bring up stomach contents that may be aspirated into the lungs, resulting in more damage to the lungs than the accident itself. If the child starts to breathe during the mouth to mouth activity, then stop the assisted breathing, but continue with the heart compressions if there is still no heartbeat or pulse. If there is a pulse or a heartbeat then stop the compressions and remain with the child until help arrives.

I would highly recommend that the primary caregiver or some other adolescent or adult, who is usually assigned to be with a child or children, undergo training in CPR (Cardio Pulmonary Resuscitation) as a precautionary measure.

NORMAL NEWBORN JAUNDICE

Jaundice is a yellow discoloration of the skin, eyes or mucus membrane and may be present at birth or at any time during the newborn period. However, there are different causes of jaundice and the management varies accordingly.

It is important to note that the physiologic or normal newborn jaundice does not pose a threat to the infant and it usually presents about the third day and disappears between 7–10 days. Every child that appears jaundiced should be seen and evaluated by a physician because one cannot diagnose any form of jaundice simply by looking at the child.

If jaundice is noted within the first twenty-four hours or after the first week of life, one can assume that it is not normal and such a child needs urgent attention. Breast-milk is sometimes associated with jaundice, but this does not mean that the child should no longer be breastfed.

Once it has been verified that the jaundice is not harmful, the treatment includes increasing the infant's feeds/fluids, exposure to sunlight or the use of special phototherapy lights. Most children do not require hospitalization and can be followed as outpatients.

If a child is noted to be greenish-yellow in appearance and appears ill, he or she should not be observed at home but should be seen and evaluated by a health-care provider because the underlying problem may be quite serious. Disorders of the liver, the digestive tract or other metabolic processes may be involved and the child may need to be hospitalized for investigations and further management.

NIGHT TERRORS

One of the most frightening experiences is being awakened in the middle of the night by a sleeping child who is screaming or making terrified sounds and movements but cannot be pacified or consoled by your efforts. Luckily this is not a very common event and usually lasts only about 10–15 minutes. This phenomenon called night terrors tends to affect children between the ages of 5–7 years, but is more common in boys than girls, and may be associated with underlying emotional problems in the child's life. The episodes usually occur between midnight and 2:00 a.m., and the child might even walk in his sleep at this time.

When a nightmare occurs the child may be easily awakened and consoled and he or she can usually say what the dream was about, however, night terrors are different in that the child cannot be aroused from the episode of terror and when he or she awakens, there is no recall. During the episode, the pupils of the eyes appear quite large, the heart rate is increased and the child breathes rapidly. This is usually followed by normal sleep and the next morning when the child awakens there is no memory of the event.

It is important to consult with the other family members when treating these children, because in most cases there are unresolved conflicts that need to be dealt with before the terrors will disappear. There might be parental discord, divorce, death or illness, peer pressure or even a new baby that may act as stress triggers for these episodes. Treatment involves family counseling and psychotherapy and for severe cases, the occasional use of medications such as Diazepam or Imipramine, for a short time period may be deemed necessary.

NOSEBLEEDS IN CHILDREN

Nosebleeds are quite common in childhood and tend to run in families. Although they may be frightening and cause parental panic, in most cases the underlying cause is neither serious nor life threatening. Bleeding is usually from the front of the nose, which has the combination of a rich blood supply and a thin protective layer.

The commonest cause is trauma from picking or rubbing the nose. Other significant causes include, inhaling dry air in the winter, insertion of a foreign body in the nose, infections of the upper respiratory tract example the common cold, sinusitis, allergic rhinitis and reflux of undigested food from the stomach up through the nostrils in young infants. In a few cases, the nosebleed may be due to a more serious problem such as a bleeding disorder, an abnormality of the blood vessels, high blood pressure, kidney disease, nasal polyps or other tumors. The use of certain drugs such as marijuana or cocaine and medications such as inhalers or nose drops for nasal congestion can also result in nosebleeds.

A healthcare provider should evaluate the child because the underlying problem may become apparent after performing a careful history and examination. An ear nose and throat specialist who will determine the need for further investigation and treatment should see children with recurrent and severe nosebleeds.

Most nosebleeds stop by themselves or they may be treated by pinching the anterior part of the nose while the child is placed in an upright or sitting position with the head tilted forward, to avoid blood trickling to the back of the throat. Other measures include the application of cold compresses, blood vessel constrictors such as Afrin. Saline nose sprays or a cool mist room humidifier may be used to prevent nosebleeds that are due to breathing dry air. A healthcare provider may be needed to treat the more persistent and recurrent cases, which might require packing the nostril and cauterizing the area with silver nitrate.

The best way to prevent nosebleeds is by finding and treating the cause. Behavior control plays a great part in avoiding the trauma due to picking and rubbing the nose.

PHENYLKETONURIA

♦

(PKU)

PKU is a disorder of the body's metabolism that occurs because of the deficiency or absence of the enzyme, phenylalanine hydroxylase, which is required to degrade the amino acid phenylalanine, to tyrosine. This results in an excessive build up of phenylalanine in the body and may lead to several problems including mental retardation.

Affected newborns appear normal at birth but if the condition is not diagnosed early they will gradually start to show symptoms such as vomiting, skin rashes, seizures and mental retardation. They usually appear blonder than their siblings, with very fair skin and blue eyes. Their heads tend to be smaller than normal and they tend to be short with small, widely spaced teeth, and prominent upper jaws. They are often described as having a mousy or musty body odor as a result of the excess phenylacetic acid in their body. Older untreated children are usually hyperactive, and exhibit abnormal involuntary movements of their limbs and bodies.

This disorder can be treated and the symptoms avoided if the diagnosis is made soon after birth. In most countries there is newborn PKU screening using the Guthrie test. This test is commonly done by piercing the heel of a newborn baby and placing the blood on a special filter paper, which is then sent to the laboratory for further testing. The test may be done as early as 4 hours after birth but it is recommended that this should be done between 48 and 72 hours. A false negative result may occur if the child has not been fed prior to the test.

The goal of treatment is to decrease the level of phenylalanine and its metabolites in the body in an effort to prevent or minimize brain damage. This is achieved by restricting the amount of phenylalanine that the child receives in his/her diet, to the minimum that is required for normal growth and development. Foods that are rich in protein are also rich in phenylalanine, therefore milk, cheese, fish, meat, poultry, eggs, legumes and nuts have to be avoided. This obviously includes a wide array of foods that are needed for normal growth; therefore there are highly specialized protein rich formula preparations that are available to ensure that these children receive a complete and balanced nutritious PKU diet. These are known as medical foods. There are different types of such foods available and they are geared toward different age groups and individual preferences. Breastfeeding may be encouraged but the phenylalanine content of the milk has to be measured and the amount of feeds regulated.

It is important to note that the blood levels of phenylalanine of affected children have to be monitored closely because of variations with growth, prolonged illness and significant changes in dietary intake. Inappropriate treatment or over-treatment in infants may result in symptoms such as lethargy, anemia, anorexia (lack of appetite), skin rashes, diarrhea and even death. One has to ensure that these children receive a diet that provides adequate calories, vitamins and other nutrients.

Dietary restriction has to continue throughout the individual's life but rigid control may be relaxed after 6 years of age. Adults who are under treated or not treated may show symptoms such as depression, anxiety, thought disorders and agoraphobia (fear of open spaces). The PKU diet may help such individuals by diminishing the severity of their symptoms. PKU can be controlled but not cured; therefore parents and children need ongoing support from highly trained and understanding healthcare personnel.

PINWORMS

Many parents can relate to the experience of being awakened by their young child early in the morning complaining about being unable to sleep because of intense itching in the area of the buttock. Many times inspection of the area may not reveal the source of the problem but it is not unreasonable to assume that he/she may be bothered by pinworms.

As the name suggests, pinworms are extremely small, about 1 cm. long, thin worms. They live in the lower parts of the intestines and during the night, the pregnant female wiggles its way down to the anus where it lays its eggs (about 11,000) before dying. The eggs are colorless and very sticky and they are the cause of the intense itching that awakens the child. Needless to say, the itching causes the child to scratch the affected area. When this occurs, the eggs get onto the fingers and under the fingernails just waiting for the opportunity to be transferred to the mouth, clothing, bedding, or another person, by the unsuspecting child. Inevitably, the eggs will eventually be transferred to the mouth, because children tend to put their fingers into their mouths quite frequently. When this occurs, the eggs are swallowed and in the stomach they hatch into small worms (larvae) that wiggle down to the lower parts of the intestines where they grow, mature and mate. The pregnant female then wiggles its way down to the anus to lay its eggs and the cycle begins all over again.

The scotch tape test is one way of detecting the eggs. This is done very early in the morning and involves pressing the sticky side of a piece of cellophane tape against the skin next to the anus, then placing it on a microscope slide with the sticky side down, followed by preservation in 75% ethyl alcohol until it can be taken to a doctor or laboratory for examination under a microscope. It is important to use gloves during the collection process because the eggs may get onto the hand of the person who is placing the tape onto the skin. Repeating the procedure on the next two days and checking other family members will yield better results. Although pinworms mainly affect children between the ages of 5 and 14 years, adults are sometimes infected.

Some doctors recommend treating everyone at home at the same time, while others, including myself, recommend treating only the ones that are infected or have symptoms. The aim is to prevent transmitting the infection from one person to another. Albendazole (Albenza) is the most highly recommended medication for killing these worms. It is taken as a single dose, by mouth and may be repeated in 2 weeks. Other effective medications include Mebendazole (Vermox) and Pyrantel Pamoate (Antiminth).

The key to prevention is to break the life cycle, because if the eggs are not swallowed they will die after about 20 days. Preventive measures include: careful hand washing before meals and after using the toilet or scratching the buttock area, avoiding sucking of the thumb or other fingers and keeping finger nails short and clean. It is also a good idea to do a thorough house cleaning at the same time by washing and drying clothes and linens, washing toilet seats, and vacuuming the bedrooms. Despite all these measures it is not unusual to have a recurrence because some eggs may have escaped during the cleaning process, some of the worms might not have been killed by the first treatment and also because there is no immunity developed to prevent having it again. Having pinworms in the family does not necessarily mean that the members are unclean and they should not be stigmatized.

PINK EYES/ CONJUNCTIVITIS

The eyes are the "windows to the soul" but when they become inflamed they feel like "the gates of hell." Anyone who has experienced having an eye infection knows that it is one of the most uncomfortable experiences in a child's life. The eyes feel as if grains of sand are sprinkled inside and they are usually itchy, red, swollen, and sometimes full of pus which cause the eyelids to become stuck with dried pus while sleeping, resulting in difficulty opening them in the morning.

It is not unusual for children to have this eye disease when they are having a cold, because they wipe their runny noses with their hands and then rub their eyes. This results in spreading of the infectious agent to the eyes. However not all cases of conjunctivitis are infectious and although the term "pink eye" is loosely used to describe inflammation of the eye that may be due to viruses, bacteria, allergens, chemicals or trauma; strictly speaking, it was originally used to refer to inflammation of the eye due to a bacterial infection. It is always better to take the child to his/her healthcare provider for evaluation, in order to receive the proper treatment and prevent possible complications.

Most cases of pink eye will respond to the soothing feel of a warm, wet washcloth that is applied to the eyes. This will also loosen up any dried pus on the eyelids, and make it easier to clean the eyes without causing further irritation. One or two drops of salt water, in the form of over the counter saline eye drops, may also relieve some of the discomfort. Your doctor will prescribe an antibiotic eye drop if there is a bacterial infection. The other forms of conjunctivitis do not require antibiotics and usually get better after a few days. The wearing of sunglasses may give some relief when the child is outdoors. Children who wear contact lenses should remove them at the first sign of inflammation, because if they continue to wear them, there could be damage to the cornea of the eye.

It is important that the child does not rub the eyes, because rubbing could introduce bacteria to an already inflamed eye and therefore result in further complications. In order to resist the urge to rub the eyes, it is a good idea to find ways of distracting the child, such as reading to him/her.

Bacterial and viral conjunctivitis are highly contagious, therefore it is important to take the necessary precautions to prevent spreading the germs from one person to the next. The easiest and best method of prevention is hand washing. Sheets, pillowcases, towels and washcloths should be washed in hot water and heat dried in an attempt to kill the offending agents.

RECURRENT ABDOMINAL PAIN

Most parents can relate to the experience of having a child with apparent abdominal discomfort and feeling absolutely helpless in affording relief. Pain in the abdomen may be reflective of problems that are producing anxiety or stress in the home, school or other aspects of the child's environment. On the other hand it could be a signal for an abdominal problem, such as appendicitis or intussusception, requiring an emergency operation.

When a child complains of pain in the abdomen, it is very important to obtain as much information as possible in an attempt to determine the underlying reason for the pain. On many occasions the source of pain may not be in the abdomen, but may be coming from the mind. When the pain is due to a particular organ disorder, the treatment is relatively simple and specific. However, when no obvious cause can be found, it can present a challenge to all concerned.

The child who experiences repeated attacks of vague, diffuse and inconsistent abdominal symptoms may need to be evaluated by a trained professional in the field of psychology. Depression, anxiety, school phobia, and emotional problems may all be manifested as abdominal pain. In these cases it is important to deal with the child in a sensitive and caring manner rather than ignore him/her and insist that nothing is wrong. Although there may be no disease in the abdomen, the pain is real and the underlying problem should be sought and dealt with before more serious manifestations appear. Children with recurrent abdominal pain ought to be evaluated by a health care professional, who should perform a thorough physical examination and have in-depth discussions with the child and the parents both together and separately, in an attempt to discover the hidden source of pain.

When there are other associated symptoms such as vomiting, fever, diarrhea, constipation, nausea, bleeding, cramping and localization, there is usually a specific organ that is inflamed or infected. These cases are not usually recurrent, and treatment may or may not require surgical intervention. It is always a good idea for the primary health care person to consult a surgeon if there is a history of sudden episodes of cramping followed by blood in the stools, because this could be indicative of a surgical emergency known as intussusception. Most people are familiar with the pain of appendicitis, which usually starts at the navel and then courses to the right mid to lower part of the abdomen. This is another surgical problem that should be addressed at the earliest opportunity. Although most cases of abdominal pain do not require surgery, it is a sad day when a child dies because of delayed intervention.

Although there are many investigations that may be performed on a child who has recurrent abdominal pain, in order to determine the proper diagnosis, it is not a good idea to over investigate these children. At times, a basic test of the stool and urine may be all that is necessary. The most effective ingredients in caring for these children include establishing an atmosphere of trust, understanding, attentiveness and genuine care and concern. This will allow the child to feel comfortable enough to open up and express the hidden emotional conflicts that are buried inside. In certain cases psychotherapy has proven to be quite valuable.

REYE'S SYNDROME

This disease was first described in 1963 by Reye and his colleagues, hence the name Reye's syndrome. It mainly affects children between the ages of 4 and 12 years of age and it is most commonly seen in those who are 6–8 years old. Boys are affected as commonly as girls are. Since the 1980's research has shown a very strong association between this disease and aspirin or medications containing acetyl salicylic acid, when taken by children who have an influenza-like illness, or chicken pox. The awareness of this association and the avoidance of these medications in susceptible children have resulted in a significant decrease in the number of cases of this disease.

Reye's syndrome consists of swelling of the brain and fatty changes in the liver. It may also affect other organs of the body, such as the kidneys, the pancreas and the heart. The degree of progression of the disease varies and one child may only have a mild case whilst another may be seriously ill to the point of actually dying. Typically, the child may have had a fever with a mild illness affecting the respiratory or gastro-intestinal systems. A few days after he/she appears to be getting better, there is a sudden onset of vomiting, weakness, drowsiness, confusion and in the more severe cases, there are seizures, abnormal posturing of the body, coma and death.

Most children are only mildly affected and they usually recover completely without any further problems. However, those that were more severely affected may later be noted to have some degree of brain damage that may be manifested in different ways, including defects in intelligence, thinking processes, visuomotor skills, abstract thinking and academic achievements.

Reye's syndrome is a potentially life-threatening disease for which there is no cure. It is important to prevent it by avoiding the use of aspirin or aspirin-like medications in children who have a fever with a flu-like illness or chicken pox.

RINGWORM

Ringworm may occur anywhere on the body but in children it is more commonly seen on the scalp than elsewhere. The name suggests that this disease is associated with a worm but it is actually caused by a fungus. It is commoner in situations of poverty and overcrowding, and mainly affects children between the ages of 4–14 years of age.

Ringworm of the scalp may present in two main ways. They are commonly known as the "black dot" and the "gray-patch" types. Although the black dot is more common than the gray patch, it is the gray patch that presents with the classical pattern, which involves one or more circular patches of broken hair on a thick, flat, scaly scalp lesion that is surrounded by a ring of reddish bumps. The black dot pattern may take a longer time to diagnose because the affected areas are quite small. Each lesion may involve only 2–3 strands of hair, which break off at the level of the scalp resulting in the appearance of a black dot on the scalp. This tends to affect a greater portion of the scalp than the gray patch type but in much smaller patches. The scalp is generally scaly and is sometimes mistaken for dandruff. These lesions are usually itchy and may become infected with bacterial organisms. When this happens, the areas tend to become raised and moist with bumps containing or oozing pus. The child might then have fever and pain, with swelling of the associated lymph glands. Depending on the severity of the condition there may be scarring with resultant permanent hair loss.

Infection may spread from one individual to another by various means. These include direct contact or contact with the infected hair and skin cells that may be present on combs, brushes, and hair ornaments or even on theater seats.

In children, ringworm of the body is most commonly acquired from contact with infected animals, such as kittens or puppies but may also be spread from scalp lesions. The most common presentation is that of a dry, reddish, scaly circular patch of skin surrounded by bumps. As the lesion enlarges, the central area appears relatively healthy whilst the borders continue to be actively involved.

Ringworm of the body sometimes heals on its own, but it responds very well to the application of antifungal creams or ointments. These include over the counter preparations that contain Miconazole (Micatin), Clotrimazole (Lotrimin) or Terbinafine (Lamisil). These agents should be applied to the affected areas twice daily for 2–4 weeks. It is usually best to continue using the cream/ointment for about 1–2 weeks after the lesion has disappeared. One should not use antibiotic or steroid containing ointments to treat these simple lesions. If there are complications such as secondary infections, then the child should be placed under the care of a competent health care provider.

Ringworm of the scalp is much more difficult to treat and the child should be seen and evaluated by a doctor prior to treatment. Therapy includes the use of an antifungal shampoo or lotion in combination with medication that has to be taken by mouth. The shampoo or lotion should contain 2.5 percent selenium sulfide (e.g. the prescription strength Selsun shampoo), Ketoconazole (Nizoral), or Zinc Pyrithione. Depending on the severity of the condition, the hair should be shampooed daily or 2–3 times each week. Your doctor may prescribe oral medication containing Griseofulvin for 2 to 12 weeks or Ketoconazole for about 1–2 weeks in selected cases. It is very important to follow your doctor's advice in order to ensure complete healing and to prevent recurrence.

Although one may not be able to prevent a child from being in contact with a playmate who has ringworm, there are measures that can be taken to decrease the chances of acquiring the infection. They should be advised against sharing hair combs, brushes and hair ornaments, hats and other objects that are in contact with the affected areas. The child may be allowed to attend school but it is a good idea to allow him/her to wear a hat or cap to cover the lesions.

RINGWORM OF THE SCALP

A fungus that invades the hair shaft resulting in hair breakage and bald patches causes ringworm of the scalp. There are different types of fungi that are associated with this illness and they present in different ways.

The child may initially have just a small bump on the scalp, which eventually spreads in a circular manner forming a red, scaly patch within which the hair becomes brittle and eventually breaks. Several bald patches may appear and they are usually quite itchy. In a few cases the body's reaction to this infection may cause the site to appear raised, boggy and weepy and may even result in permanent baldness and scarring.

The fungus is highly contagious and is usually spread by contact with infected hair or skin. This may be by sharing hats, combs, brushes, scrungies or other hair ornaments or by placing one's head on surfaces such as benches, chairs or even theater seats. In rare instances, the disease may be acquired from contact with pets such as cats and dogs.

Patients should be seen by a healthcare professional who will prescribe a medication that is taken by mouth for 4–16 weeks, but usually an average of 6 weeks. The patient is also advised to use special shampoos that will decrease the scaliness of the scalp and shorten the length of time that the individual is at risk of spreading the infection. It is important to note that the shampoos neither cure nor shorten the course of the illness.

ROSEOLA

Roseola is one of the viral diseases of childhood that is usually quite puzzling for both the parents and the physician in its early stages, but it becomes really easy to diagnose as the illness progresses. It is more commonly seen during the spring and fall months but it may occur at any time.

In the early stages, children with Roseola appear to be generally well apart from the fact that they have a fever. Typically the fever tends to be relatively high, ranging from 101–106^{oF} (37.9–40.0^{oC}), and after 3–5 days it suddenly disappears. Within 12–24 hours of the breaking of the fever, a rosy, pink rash appears. This rash usually starts on the trunk of the body and then quickly spreads to the neck, face and upper parts of the limbs. There is no associated itching and it generally disappears after 1–3 days. If the child is uncomfortable or if the fever is over 102^{oF}, it is a good idea to give these children some fever reducing medication. This will relieve the discomfort caused by the fever and is also a precautionary measure for the minority of children who may develop febrile seizures as a complication. Fever reducing medications containing acetaminophen or ibuprofen are recommended. Aspirin should be avoided due to its association with the development of brain and liver damage (Reye's syndrome) when taken by some children who have viral illnesses. In order to avoid dehydration they should be encouraged to drink a lot of fluid.

The Roseola virus is usually transmitted from one person to another via saliva and can occur in children at anytime. This is a relatively mild illness and currently there are no vaccines or any specific ways to prevent it.

ROCKY MOUNTAIN SPOTTED FEVER

Enjoying the outdoors is not without danger as evidenced by the fact that the majority of cases of Rocky Mountain spotted fever occur during April through October and in children aged 5–9 years. Initially it may be difficult to diagnose because the child may have non-specific symptoms such as headache, fever, muscle pains, lack of appetite, restlessness, vomiting, diarrhea, nausea and abdominal pains. However after about 3 days the typical rash appears that brings some clarity to the overall picture. The rash often begins as a small area of pale, rose-red spots on the ankles, wrists or lower legs but rapidly spreads to involve the entire body, even the palms and soles. After a few days, it begins to look redder and sometimes there are areas that appear to be bruised. As the disease progresses, the initial symptoms tend to get worse and there may even be severe damage to any one of the organs in the body. This includes the liver, kidneys, lungs, spleen, heart and brain. Failure of any of these organs could result in the death of the child.

This disease is caused by an organism named Rickettsia Rickettsii that is injected into the skin whenever an infected tick bites an individual. This tick may be present on dogs and other small mammals that are in contact with humans as they explore the outdoors. In most cases the tick bite goes unnoticed and the illness simply appears. If one is lucky enough to notice the tick during its feeding episode it is best to remove it by pulling it slowly and steadily from as close to the skin surface as possible, with an instrument such as a pair of tweezers. Never touch the tick with bare hands and never attempt to kill it by slapping it with the palm of the hand, as we usually do to kill mosquitoes.

If the diagnosis is made and treatment is started within the first 3 days of the illness, the child will begin to improve within 24–72 hours with complete recovery within 7–10 days. However if treatment is delayed, severe complications could result in coma and death. The child must be seen by a healthcare professional who will prescribe one or more antibiotics such as Chloramphenicol, Doxycycline or Tetracycline. Tetracycline might cause permanent staining of the teeth in children less than 8 years old, but if there is no alternative, the short course used is relatively safe.

There are no vaccines available to prevent this disease but several precautionary measures may be taken to decrease the chances of being bitten by an infected tick when enjoying the pleasures of the outdoors. These include wearing clothing that covers the legs and arms, using insect repellent, making frequent inspections for ticks (it may take hours for a tick to feed and cause an infection) and not touching it with the bare hands.

SCOLIOSIS

Many parents have noticed that their pre-adolescent children tend to slouch and at times their spines appear to be twisted, giving an s-shaped appearance. This may be due to a condition known as scoliosis. There are different causes of scoliosis, ranging from those children that are born with a spinal deformity or damage to the brain (congenital), to those who develop it later in life, for no apparent reason (idiopathic). The congenital cases of scoliosis tend to be more severe and more progressive than the idiopathic ones. There are some children who have one leg that is a little shorter than the other and this may result in a mild tilting of the pelvis that gives a scoliotic appearance.

Girls are affected more frequently than boys and the condition is more likely to get worse if there is significant curving before the onset of the first period in girls and before the voice change in boys. In the United States of America most cases are detected in the middle school years when routine scoliosis screening is performed at school. Not all cases will require special treatment such as bracing or even surgery, but all cases should be followed and investigated by their physician. Some children may require only observation every 6–12 months because the majority will straighten up as they grow. Others, however, may need special x-rays and further referral to a bone specialist (Orthopedic surgeon). The main reasons for identifying and treating these children as early as possible include: prevention of further deformity, prevention of damage to the affected joints, prevention of certain disorders of the lung and heart as well as the obviously negative impact on the child's self image.

Although different methods of treatment have been tried, there is no proof that exercise or electrical stimulation have affected the outcome of children with progressive scoliosis. Bracing remains quite popular but its long-term effect remains questionable. Surgical correction is undoubtedly the best method for severe cases.

It is extremely important to encourage these children and not to make an issue about their disorder because they are at the age where they are trying to discover their identity and are easily embarrassed and feel ostracized whenever they appear to be different from their peers. Positive reinforcement is the key ingredient to helping them achieve self-esteem and overcoming this awkward stage of their development.

SEIZURES DUE TO FEVER

◆

(FEBRILE SEIZURES)

One of the most distressing events that parents have to endure is to see their child having a seizure. About 3–4% of young children will have a seizure that is triggered by a high fever. It tends to occur in children between 9 months and 5 years, but is most often seen in children between 14–18 months of age. There is a strong tendency for this condition to run in families and the good news is that it usually disappears as the child gets older. The seizure itself is not usually harmful to the child, and the most common underlying reason for the fever is a viral infection of the ear or the respiratory tract. However, it is of paramount importance that the child is seen and evaluated for any serious infection such as meningitis or infection of the blood stream (sepsis) that could have very serious consequences if they are not treated early. Most febrile seizures are of short duration, lasting a few seconds to a maximum of about 10 minutes. They usually occur when the body's temperature rises rapidly to a level that is equal to or higher than 39^{oc} ($102\ ^{oF}$). The typical pattern of this type of seizure is that the entire body is affected, in that there is loss of consciousness and the child's body becomes rigid before the arms and legs begin to contract in spasms. There is usually drooling from the mouth, the eyes tend to roll over, and there may or may not be loss of control of the muscles of the anus and the bladder resulting in involuntary soiling and passing of urine. At the end of the episode there is some drowsiness.

A simple febrile seizure has certain characteristics that include the following: it does not usually last longer than 15 minutes, it does not affect only one side of the body and it does not usually recur after a few hours or days in the absence of a fever. If any of these occur, the child should be investigated for other underlying problems, which include epilepsy, electrolyte imbalances, infantile spasms and brain tumors.

The main points to remember when a child is having a seizure are:

- Keep the airway open, by holding the head slightly backward with the chin in an upward position. Do not place anything in the mouth such as a spoon or a finger.

- Do not panic.

- Do not leave the child unattended.

- Call for help (911).

- Prevent injuries to the child.

- Remove blankets or other such covers.

- Try cooling the child by sponging him or her with tepid water. (Not alcohol).

- Do not try to stop the seizure by holding the limbs.

- Be patient. The seizure will eventually stop within a few seconds or minutes.

After the seizure has stopped and the child is awake and alert, give him or her some fever reducing medication such as acetaminophen (Tylenol or ibuprofen (Advil, Motrin). Do not give aspirin, because of its association with the development of Reye's syndrome.

Febrile seizures may recur; therefore a child who has had one episode should be closely watched whenever he or she has a fever. It is wise to give such a child a fever reducing medicine at the onset of a fever and to keep him or her as cool as possible. These children should be seen and evaluated shortly after they develop an illness that is accompanied by a fever, even if it is only a mild cold. It is reassuring to note that these seizures do not cause brain damage and the children can live and learn like other children without any need for specific medication for the seizures.

SEIZURES NOT DUE TO FEVER

✦

(EPILEPSY)

A seizure is a symptom that lets one know that something is wrong inside the brain, and although all epileptic attacks are seizures, not all seizures are epilepsy. In fact, as long as there is a specific underlying problem such as fever, infection of the brain or its coverings, trauma or electrolyte imbalance that results in the seizure, the condition is not considered to be epilepsy. To further clarify the situation, the term epilepsy is not applied until there are two or more of these non-febrile seizures. About 3–5% of children have seizures, while less than 1.0% have epilepsy.

There are different forms of epilepsy and most children will have the same type each time that they have an episode, but there are times when one child will have a mixture of the different types. The mixed ones are usually more difficult to treat. Epilepsy tends to run in families and on a lot of occasions, the cause is not known.

Most people are familiar with the "grand mal" seizure, which is associated with loss of consciousness, abnormal jerky movements and stiffening of the entire body. However, seizures may appear as a brief episode of staring in space, sudden stiffening out of all or part of the body, sudden loss of body tone resulting in a fall, sudden jerking of all or part of the body, or a combination of these with or without loss of consciousness. It is very important to describe the seizure as accurately as possible to your healthcare provider, because the management varies depending on the type of seizure. In most instances it is the history of the event that assists in making the diagnosis and not investigations such as EEG (electro-encephalogram) and CT scans, because the results of these tests may be normal between the seizure episodes.

The main points to remember when a child is having a seizure are:

- Keep the airway open, by holding the head slightly backward with the chin in an upward position. Do not place anything in the mouth such as a spoon or a finger.

- Do not panic.

- Do not leave the child unattended.

- Call for help (911).

- Prevent injuries to the child.

- Do not try to stop the seizure by holding the limbs.

- Be patient. The seizure will eventually stop within a few seconds or minutes.

Children who have epilepsy will require medication for a prolonged period of time and generally they have to be without seizures for about two years before the decision is made to gradually stop the medication. It is very important that the child is evaluated and followed up closely by their health care provider because these medicines may sometimes have undesirable side effects.

SICKLE CELL ANEMIA

Sickle cell anemia receives its name from the shape of the red blood cells that are affected by this disorder. The sickle hemoglobin (HbS) is different from normal adult hemoglobin because of a mutation that results in the substitution of the amino acid Glutamic acid, by another amino acid Valine, at the sixth position of the beta hemoglobin chain. In situations where the amount of oxygen in the circulation is deficient, the affected red cells become rigid, brittle, and insoluble. This results in stacks of sickled red cells obstructing the blood flow, which in turn causes a decrease in oxygen to the affected area, thereby causing further sickling and perpetuating a vicious cycle. Damage to the red cell membrane shortens its life span and results in an anemia that is called hemolytic anemia. This may cause the individual to have gallstones, appear pale, jaundiced (yellow eyes), easily tired, and not able to achieve his/her growth potential.

There are newborn screening programs that are implemented in most parts of the world that are used to detect the presence of sickled cells at birth. DNA testing can detect this disorder even before the child is born. Affected babies may appear normal at birth and the earliest sign may be pallor, due to anemia, showing up between 2 to 4 months of age. The first obvious symptom usually presents between 5 to 6 months of age as painful swellings of the hands and feet. This is called the "hand-foot syndrome" or sickle dactylitis.

The sickled cells may cause obstruction of blood flow to different areas of the body, resulting in the presentation of different crises. These are intermittent episodic events that tend to occur in children. Some of the serious and more common crises include:

- Bone infarction—causing severe bone pain with or without swelling.

- Splenic sequestration—causing sudden pooling of blood in the spleen that can result in shock and death.

- Blocked brain blood vessels/stroke—causing bleeding or infarction in the brain that may result in weakness or paralysis of the affected parts of the body.

- Acute chest syndrome—causing severe chest pain which may be due to infarction or infection i.e. Pneumonia. In some instances these patients require assisted breathing with a mechanical ventilator.

- Repeated splenic infarctions—causing loss of function of the spleen, which results in the individual's inability to fight certain infections and the possibility of an early death.

- Blocked kidney vessels—causing an inability to concentrate the urine, blood in the urine and damage to parts of the kidney, which may result in kidney failure and death.

Most patients with this disease may remain relatively well for long periods of time and it is of paramount importance to educate them and their parents about how to check for early warning signs of a severe crisis and how to avoid factors that may bring on a crisis.

It is important that these children drink adequate amount of fluids to prevent dehydration and they should not over-exert themselves with strenuous physical exercise. They should avoid cold temperatures, alcohol abuse, and exercising at high altitudes. They need to know their normal/steady state hemoglobin levels, which are usually between 5 and 9 g/dl. Parents should be aware that fever should not be ignored and the child with a fever should be promptly seen and evaluated by a trained medical individual.

Children must be fully immunized and in addition they should also receive the Pneumococcal polyvalent vaccine at age 2 years with boosters at ages 5 and 10 years. Hepatitis B vaccine and H. Influenzae vaccines are also indicated. In an attempt to prevent serious infections, children below the age of 5 years or those above 5 years who have had their spleen removed or have had several Pneumococcal bacterial infections, should be maintained on Penicillin V given twice daily by mouth.

Most painful episodes may be managed out of the hospital setting and one has to be careful about giving narcotics such as Pethidine because some patients may develop a dependency on these drugs. These children should not be given iron supplements unless blood investigations deem it necessary, because they may develop complications from having excess iron in their bodies. Blood transfusions are rarely indicated and only for very specific instances such as prior to major surgery or for severe splenic sequestration crises.

SINUSITIS

Most of us are familiar with the constant dripping of a faulty tap and at best it can be described as being one of the most annoying things that we might have to deal with in life. This is basically what the individual with sinusitis has to endure when the sinuses are inflamed, because fluid drips downward from the sinuses to the back of the throat causing the child to cough, sniff, snort, swallow, clear his or her throat and to have a runny nose on an on-going basis.

The sinuses are groups of air cells that develop from the lining of the nose and are located in the areas of the forehead, the cheeks and around the eyes. They all have tubes that drain into the nose; therefore if the nostrils are blocked for any reason, the sinuses may become inflamed and produce the symptoms of sinusitis. Allergic symptoms such as allergic rhinitis and infections such as the common cold commonly occur before an attack of sinusitis. However, other factors that may trigger sinusitis include exposure to cigarette smoking, inhaling cold or dry air, swimming, reflux of food from the stomach, facial trauma or injuries, disorders of the immune system and the genes (eg.cystic fibrosis), enlarged adenoids, and tumors such as nasal polyps.

Although adolescents and adults commonly complain of headaches, pain, tenderness and swelling of the face, younger children do not usually develop these symptoms. The commonest symptoms in children are a runny nose, a sore throat and a cough that seems to get worse at nights or when the child is lying on the back. Sometimes they may have a decreased sense of smell, a feeling of pressure on the face, fever, or even a "bad breath" that does not disappear with proper brushing of the teeth.

It is important that the child is seen and evaluated by a health care professional so that the necessary investigations and treatment can be started at the earliest opportunity. Complications may arise as a result of spreading of the infection to nearby structures including the middle ear, eyes, brain (meningitis or abscess), and bone (osteomyelitis). Most children will recover when they are given antibiotics, such as Amoxicillin, Augmentin, Cefuroxime or Erythromycin for 10–14 days. Using salt-water nose sprays and decongestants may give some relief, but they do not make the child get better any faster. Antihistamines may cause thickening of the secretions and therefore could make the sinusitis worse, therefore they are not recommended. If the child develops complications affecting the eyes or the brain, he or she may have to be admitted to the hospital for more intensive treatment. In rare instances, surgical treatment including sinus aspiration may be recommended for cases that do not respond to standard therapy.

SPRAINS AND STRAINS

Sprains and strains can occur wherever there are muscles and joints in the body. However most of us are familiar with these injuries occurring at the ankles. They both present with pain and swelling due to injury to the soft tissues, rather than bone. Therefore it is sometimes difficult to determine whether the problem is a strain or a sprain.

A sprain is the term used to describe what occurs when a ligament or a joint capsule is torn or stretched whilst a strain describes injury to a muscle and its tendon. In its simplest form one may say that a strain is mainly associated with a muscle injury while a sprain is mainly associated with a joint injury. ("Strain a muscle and sprain a joint").

The wearing of high-top shoes and the use of an ankle brace may decrease the chances of receiving an ankle injury; however taping the ankle with adhesive tape does not provide adequate support for injury prevention. Most of these injuries are minor and heal without complications, however there are a few that may be serious enough to require surgical repair. Therefore it is always better to seek medical advice when these injuries occur.

The management of these conditions is based on the same principles; therefore one need not focus too much on whether the injury is a strain or a sprain. The treatment involves Rest, Ice, Compression and Elevation. Think of RICE and you should be able to remember what to do.

Rest: The affected area should be rested for the first 2–3 days. If it's the ankle, the child should not be allowed to stand, walk or bear the body's weight. This will help to prevent further injury to the area as well as decrease the amount of pain.

Ice: Ice chips or ice water should be placed on the affected area as soon as possible and be kept there for at least 20 minutes. This should be repeated 2–4 times per day for the first 2–3 days. The ice causes the blood vessels to get smaller so that there is less bleeding, pain and swelling. Do not use heat because it will make the situation worse.

Compression: An elastic bandage should be applied firmly and evenly to the area, but it should not be too tight because the blood supply might be affected. The bandage should be removed immediately if the child complains of discomfort or if the area below the bandage looks pale or blue. The pressure decreases the amount of swelling and the associated pain that may occur. It is always better if the bandage is applied by a healthcare professional.

Elevation: Whenever possible, the affected area should be raised above the level of the heart. This will decrease the amount of swelling because it will improve the blood flow away from the affected area.

Shortly after the injury, measures should be taken to start rehabilitating the affected area. This should be done in a slow and organized manner. Initially one should concentrate on recovering the normal range of motion by passive then by active therapy, followed by strengthening, endurance and agility exercises. When the child is able to comfortably perform all the normal activities associated with the affected area, then one may assume that healing is complete. Full recovery is required to prevent recurrent injuries. If discomfort persists after 9–12 months of satisfactory rehabilitation, the patient should be re-evaluated by an orthopedic surgeon.

STREP THROAT/SORE THROAT

✦

(STREPTOCOCCAL PHARYNGITIS)

It is very common to hear someone say that his or her child has a "strep throat," but it is not unusual to find that most people do not really understand the significance of this disease. The term "strep" refers to the bacteria described as group A beta hemolytic streptococcus, and its main danger is the possible development of acute rheumatic fever following a throat infection. It is often present in the 5–15 age groups and is uncommon in children less than 2 years of age.

It is important to note that most sore throats are due to viral infections and that it is not possible to merely look at the throat of an ill child and diagnose the causal agent. Your health care provider will take a swab of your child's throat and perform a rapid test for the streptococcus organism and may also send a specimen to the laboratory for culture. Generally speaking, the child with a viral throat infection may have other symptoms such as a runny nose, runny eyes, cough, hoarseness, diarrhea, or a skin rash before the throat begins to hurt. On the other hand, the child with a "strep throat" may complain of a headache, fever, pain in the abdomen, and may even vomit before the throat becomes a problem. The sore throat may cause mild to severe pain on swallowing and the lymph glands in the neck may become swollen and tender. The throat usually appears red and the tonsils may or may not be enlarged. The fever usually lasts for 1–4 days, but the symptoms may persist for a longer period if the child is severely ill. If left untreated, the disease could either get better on its own or spread to involve the ears (otitis media), sinuses (sinusitis), or the brain (meningitis). An immune reaction in the body sometimes follows a "strep throat" and may result in rheumatic fever, which could damage the heart (rheumatic carditis) or infection of the kidneys (post streptococcal glomerulonephritis).

103

Once it has been determined that a child has a "strep throat," he or she should be given antibiotics, such as Penicillin or Amoxicillin for 10 days. Gargling with warm salt water or taking painkillers such as Ibuprofen (Motrin) or Acetaminophen (Tylenol) may relieve the pain in the throat. Young children may also get some pain relief from steam inhalation. It is important to encourage the child to drink a lot of fluids in order to prevent dehydration, but he or she might resist because of the pain that is associated with swallowing. Cool, non-acidic drinks, such as ginger ale may be well tolerated. The child should not be forced to eat solids at this time.

This disease is contagious and can be passed on to others by sharing drinking or eating utensils, kissing, coughing, and sharing objects that have been placed in the mouth of an infected child. However, this ability to infect others disappears after a few hours of starting antibiotic treatment. As mentioned before, the main danger lies in the complications and not the throat infection itself.

SUDDEN INFANT DEATH SYNDROME

◆

(SIDS)

Sudden infant death syndrome (SIDS), as the name suggests, occurs suddenly, without warning or explanation and causes profound grief that is compounded by unanswered questions and a lot of guilt and self blame. Although it is quite a common cause of death in infants between the ages of 1 month to 1 year, with the majority occurring between 2 to 4 months, the exact cause still remains a mystery.

Prematurity and a low birth weight appear to be common factors among victims of SIDS, and other associated factors include the use of drugs such as methadone, heroin, nicotine and cocaine by the pregnant mother. Children who have had a sister or brother die of SIDS are also at increased risk of a similar death.

Studies have shown that the underlying problem appears to be an abnormality in the part of the brain that is responsible for controlling the link between breathing and the beating of the heart. When there is not enough oxygen getting to the brain, instead of the heart rate increasing, or the infant waking up to gasp for air, the rate actually slows down and then the heart eventually stops beating. It is not yet clear why this occurs and unfortunately, there is no real test available to detect which child will die of SIDS and which one will not, before it actually happens.

However, there are certain precautions that can be taken to protect children against SIDS: these include placing infants on their back when they go to sleep, avoiding soft bedding, pillows, comforters, duvets, covers over the infant's head, and bed sharing. The use of home monitors and surveillance cameras may assist in preventing death in some cases but they have not proven to be as effective as was previously hoped.

SUNBURN AND SKIN CANCER

Children enjoy being outdoors where they are able to run and play freely and explore the wonders of nature. However, exposure to the ultra-violet rays of the sun may damage the skin and may at times result in skin cancer. It is therefore very important to apply sweat proof and waterproof sunscreens to your child's skin before he or she goes out to play or swim.

Children below the age of 2 years need to be protected with sunscreens that have a sun protective factor (SPF) of 8–15, whilst those over age 2 years require those with a SPF of at least 15. Light cotton clothing and hats, caps or sun visors are also recommended for the outdoors. All skin types are susceptible to being burnt by the sun, but children with very pale skin, light eyes and hair color, are extremely susceptible to the damaging effects of the ultraviolet rays of the sun. A sure sign of too much exposure to the sun is the appearance of freckles. The practice of exposing oneself to the sun in order to get tanned is dangerous and should be discouraged. Skin cancer is so common and deadly that it now accounts for the death of one American each hour.

Not all cases of skin cancer are due to sun exposure, but the majority is, therefore it is prudent to prevent this avoidable disease by dressing appropriately and applying sunscreens before going outdoors during the hot months of spring and summer. It is important to note that even in some areas where snow sports are popular, the rays of the sun are still quite damaging, and therefore protective measures need to be taken. Tanning salons also pose a risk for the development of skin cancer and children should not be allowed to utilize these facilities.

SWIMMER'S EAR AND OUTER EAR INFECTIONS IN CHILDREN

Although swimmer's ear is the term used to describe this condition, it may occur in the absence of swimming. Excessive moisture, dryness, skin disorders such as eczema or dermatitis and trauma may affect the normal skin barrier in such a way that the resistance to infection is decreased. A child who has an infection of the outer ear usually presents with itching followed by pain, swelling and redness of the affected area. There may or may not be pus draining from the ear canal and the usual golden brown wax may be replaced by a soft, whitish material. In long-standing or severe cases, there may be mild hearing loss. It is very important that a child with this problem is seen, evaluated and treated by a health care professional in the early stages. Failure to do so may result in complications. These include; weakness or paralysis of the nerves in the affected area, deafness, and spreading of the infection to the nearby bone and the base of the skull.

Most cases will respond to ear drops or ointments that contain antibiotics and a steroid preparation. Several home remedies have proven to be effective in reducing the swelling and pain in uncomplicated cases. These include the application of 2% Acetic acid (vinegar) or half-strength Burrow's solution. Dry heat as well as painkillers containing Ibuprofen may be required in the more severe cases. If there is an associated fever and swelling of the lymph glands in the area, antibiotics will be needed. It is a good idea for your health care provider to obtain a swab of the infectious material for laboratory identification of the offending organism, although one does not have to wait for the results before starting treatment. Quite frequently there may be a mixture of bacteria and even fungi growing in the ear canal. Anti-fungal medications including 2% Gentian Violet, Nystatin or Clotrimazole are needed for cases that are associated with fungi, because antibiotics will not be effective.

Children who do a lot of swimming are prone to getting repeated infections of the outer ear. They may be able to decrease the number of recurrences by placing

107

drops of dilute alcohol or 2% Acetic acid into the ear canal immediately after swimming or bathing. A child who has an outer ear infection should not be allowed to swim and water should not be allowed to get into the infected ear during bathing.

TEETHING

The appearance of an infant's first tooth is an exciting milestone that usually occurs between 6 and 8 months of age. Although some babies have no significant discomfort, the majority have associated pain, irritability, swollen, sensitive gums, and excessive drooling. If a baby has vomiting, diarrhea, fever, rash or runny nose at the time that they are teething, it is important to note that teething is not responsible for the symptoms and they are only coincidental findings. One should never attribute a high fever to teething, but should remember that at this age babies are at risk of being infected with viruses and bacteria. During the teething period they tend to put their fingers and other objects in their mouths, and this behavior places them at an even higher risk of getting an infection. One should not delay taking an ill infant for an evaluation by a healthcare professional, simply because he or she is teething.

The mainstay of caring for these infants is to provide relief for their aching gums. Most babies respond favorably to biting on a cool, firm object such as a cooled teething ring, a wet wash cloth or ice wrapped in cloth. Teething rusks or biscuits can be helpful but may cause choking due to their tendency to crumble. Pain medications containing Acetaminophen or Ibuprofen may allow the baby to feed and sleep more comfortably. There are several over the counter anesthetic gels, such as Orajel and Ambesol, which are used to make the gums less sensitive. I have found it very difficult to apply the gel only to the affected areas in a crying, irritable baby, but some parents have reported good results. As babies get older they appear to have less discomfort, therefore time, patience and tender loving care are key ingredients in caring for them.

There are a few babies who are born with one or more teeth. These teeth may represent the primary teeth which have erupted in the womb or they may be extra teeth that might prevent the proper eruption of the primary teeth. When this happens it is a good idea to consult with a dental surgeon who may or may not recommend extraction after reviewing the relevant x-rays. Sometimes there are clear swellings on the gum that may be mistaken for teeth, these are cystic lesions that will eventually disappear and require no special treatment. Being born with teeth does not mean that the baby is abnormal and does not mean that he or she will have developmental problems.

TENSION/STRESS HEADACHES

Many adults think that the stresses and anxieties that children face on an ongoing basis do not affect them. However, nothing could be further from the truth. Their anger or frustrations may be manifested as headaches, abdominal pain, bed-wetting, constipation or even eating disorders. Tension headaches are more commonly found in the pre-adolescent age group and tend to occur during periods of stress, such as school examinations, family conflicts, divorce, relocation, peer pressure or death of a family member or a close friend.

Unlike migraine, the headache is not usually throbbing and is mainly described as a feeling of pressure or tightening of the scalp. It may be localized in the front, the top or the back of the head and there may be tenderness of the affected area. There is no associated nausea or vomiting as would be expected in a child who has migraine or a brain tumor. Most children can figure out the underlying cause of their headaches and will divulge it if they are placed in a setting that makes them feel comfortable enough to discuss their concerns.

A child who has recurrent tension headaches should be evaluated and carefully examined by their health care provider. The diagnosis does not usually require extensive investigations such as x-rays, CT scans (Computerized Tomography), or MRI (Magnetic Resonance Imaging). Several pointers include a poor self-image, fear of school failure, lack of self-confidence, and lack of friends. The affected children may appear depressed and exhibit mood swings, weight gain or loss, eating disorders, disturbed sleep, fatigue and withdrawal from social activities. Management mainly involves a search for underlying emotional and stressful factors followed by reassurance and explanation of how stress produces headaches by causing a constant contraction of certain muscles in the region of the head and neck. In most cases, over the counter painkillers such as acetaminophen (Tylenol), or ibuprofen (Motrin) may be beneficial. Severe cases may require a brief period of hospitalization in order to remove the child from the stressful environment and observe how he or she interacts with other people. In many instances, the headache resolves without further medication whilst in others self-relaxation techniques and biofeedback are required.

Regardless of the severity, these children should be dealt with on an individual basis and their needs and concerns met in a caring and non-threatening environment. The child should be evaluated and provisions made for individual and family counseling sessions by trained psychotherapists, as well as emotional and moral support from school personnel and family members.

THRUSH

Most parents are familiar with the milky coating that tends to build up on our baby's tongue after feeding and know that a drink of water or a gentle wipe with a soft, moist cloth will remove it. There are times however, when these simple measures do not work and the coating just seems to get worse and spread to the gums and even the corners of the mouth. One might even see mild bleeding when attempts are made to scrape off the coating. It is usually at this point that some mothers seek professional advice and are told that their baby has thrush.

This is an infection that is caused by a fungus and affects 2–5% of normal newborn babies. The fungus lives in the mother's vaginal area and gets into the baby's mouth as it passes through the birth canal. The baby's immune system is immature at this time and the fungus therefore gets an opportunity to grow and multiply in the baby's mouth where the environment is ideal, being warm, dark, sweet and moist. Although it may occur in healthy newborns, it is often seen in babies whose immune system is rendered even more deficient because of other illnesses such as HIV, the virus that causes AIDS or more commonly, antibiotic therapy that was prescribed for a bacterial infection.

The baby may not show any discomfort from the infection but when there is a heavy coating of this curdy material, it may cause pain, fussiness and decreased feeding. Treatment is quite simple and babies usually show improvement shortly after starting the anti-fungal medication. The most popular treatment is Nystatin suspension that is placed in the mouth four times per day after feeding; however there are more effective medications which include Miconazole gel, Amphotericin B suspension, and Gentian Violet. Although the coating might disappear after a few days, it is important to continue treatment for 7–10 days to avoid a relapse.

TOILET TRAINING

Toilet training should not be a stressful process for you or your child and it is of paramount importance that too much emphasis is not placed on this event. The age of readiness varies but generally boys tend to be ready at a later age than girls. Most children are able to verbalize their toilet desires at about 18–24 months. In the United States, the average age for achieving toilet training is 27 months but the normal range extends to 3–4 years. The child usually shows his or her readiness either by removing the soiled pants or by voicing discomfort. He or she may also be able to hold back the desire for a short while on request.

Toddler "potties" are effective for initial training and as the child grows, they may be allowed to use training "potties" on the adult's toilet until he or she is tall and large enough to actually sit on the toilet seat without the risk of falling inside the bowl. Parents can use their imagination when encouraging a child to use the "potty." They can create games such as the color change scenario where the child can magically change the blue water in the toilet bowl to green by simply passing urine into the bowl. They may also be rewarded each time they are successful in getting to the potty before the actual elimination process begins. They should not be "shamed" or ostracized when they fail and too much emphasis should not be placed on this event.

Everyone eventually learns the behaviors that are accepted by their society and parents should be patient and not be overly concerned about their child mastering a skill at a certain specified age. There is really no need to have the child accompany an adult into the bathroom to observe what he or she does whenever they urinate or defecate. There is no research to show that this will hasten the training process. Trying to train a child who is not yet ready will result in anger, frustration and even ultimately personality problems. Gentle persuasion and praise are the keys to success.

UMBILICAL CARE

The umbilicus or navel represents the remnants of the source of nutrition and blood circulation between the fetus and the mother while the child was inside the womb. At the time of birth this cord is cut and has to be kept clean in order to prevent the development of an infection. It is highly recommended that the cord should be cleaned with alcohol swabs at the time of each diaper change. The use of triple dye or antibiotic ointments may be recommended in certain cases of mild infection. Sloughing and healing are usually complete within two weeks. Some parents are afraid of touching the cord or even allowing it to get wet. Such fear is unfounded and if we remember that the baby was suspended in fluid inside the womb then this will support the fact that it is perfectly safe to allow water to be in contact with the cord during the baby's baths.

Quite often healing is delayed because of a pink, fleshy overgrowth of tissue at the base of the umbilicus. This is called a granuloma and it can be easily treated with one or more applications of silver nitrate. Many newborns have a protuberant umbilicus or hernia, however most of these disappear by two years of age and even very large ones sometimes disappear by 5 to 6 years. There is absolutely nothing to be gained by "strapping the navel." There is no evidence that it prevents the child from having an "outtie" and it may actually result in abdominal discomfort and breathing difficulties.

The infant should be seen and evaluated by a pediatrician if there is swelling and or redness surrounding the umbilicus or if the cord has not sloughed off after one month. These signs may be due to an infection or an underlying medical problem. If urine or feces is noted to be coming from the umbilicus, it means that the infant has a serious underlying problem and he or she will require surgical intervention.

URINARY TRACT INFECTIONS

✦

(UTI's)

The urinary tract may become infected from below or above the bladder and it is not uncommon for little girls to develop this complication around the time when they are trying to master their bowel habits. It is very important to teach them to wipe from front to back after passing stool because to do otherwise may cause the introduction of bacteria from the anal region to the urethra that opens just in front of the vagina. The urethra is a narrow tube that comes from the bladder and forms the passage through which urine flows out of the body. During the first year of life uncircumcised boys appear to be at an increased risk of getting this infection, because bacteria may collect under the foreskin and then make their way into the urethra which opens at the tip of the penis. Due to the close relationship of the openings of the urethra and the anus, UTI's are more common in females than in males.

Infection may involve the bladder, or lower part of the urinary tract (cystitis) or the kidneys, or upper portion (pyelitis, pyelonephritis) or both. Infection of the kidneys is much more serious than that of the bladder. However, bladder infection can produce a backward flow of urine, which could result in infection and damage to the kidneys. Repeated episodes of infection may result in scarring of the kidneys and that could lead to high blood pressure and kidney failure. It is therefore very important to have the child seen and evaluated as early as possible by a healthcare provider who will obtain a sample of urine for urinalysis and culture, before starting treatment.

The symptoms vary with the age and location of the infection. Babies often present with a variety of symptoms including: jaundice, diarrhea, vomiting, fussiness, fever, poor feeding, and loss of weight. Bladder infection in the older child may result in complaints of burning and increased frequency of passing urine, bedwetting and urinary accidents during the daytime, pain in the lower part of the abdomen and the urine may have an unpleasant odor or may even appear cloudy or blood stained. Boys may sometimes notice that they have difficulty passing a full and strong stream of urine. When the kidney is infected, the symptoms may include: pain in one or both sides of the abdomen, fever, nausea, vomiting, diarrhea, loss of appetite and a general feeling of being unwell.

Most children with infection of the lower urinary tract will recover after receiving a 3–5 day course of antibiotics such as Trimethoprim-Sulphamethoxazole/TMP-SMZ (Septra, Cotrim, Bactrim), Nitrofurantoin, or Amoxicillin (Amoxil). Infection of the upper urinary tract requires treatment for about 14 days and in some cases the child may have to be admitted to hospital.

If the illness is mild, the child may be given only oral antibiotics. For more severe cases a combination of both oral and injected antibiotics may be given in order to ensure that the level of antibiotics in the body is high enough to destroy the bacteria before they cause complications. It is a good idea to repeat the urine culture about 1 week after the end of treatment and periodically during the next 1–2 years.

There are certain precautions that may be taken to prevent first or repeated attacks of UTI's. Included among these are:

- Encouraging frequent trips to the bathroom to pass urine, rather than holding back and resisting the urge.

- Drinking about 8 glasses (8 ounces each) of water each day.

- Encouraging regular passing of stool, to prevent constipation, which may cause UTI's.

- Adding cranberry juice to the diet, in order to change the pH to an alkaline range thus discouraging the growth and multiplication of bacteria.

- Taking low dose antibiotics such as TMP-SMZ (Septra) or Amoxicillin to prevent repeated attacks.

- Encouraging girls to wipe from front to back rather than back to front, after using the toilet.

- Avoiding frequent bubble baths.

- Avoiding tight-fitting pants and underwear.

- Treating for pinworms if present.

Although UTI's are curable, as with any infection, it is much better to take the necessary steps toward prevention rather than trying to effect a cure.

REFERENCES

Nelson, Textbook of Pediatrics, Behrman, Kliegman, Jenson, 16 th Edition

Gellis & Kagan's, Current Pediatric Therapy, W.B. Saunders, Harcourt Brace, 14th International Edition

Behrman, Kliegman, Jenson, "Nelson Textbook of Pediatrics" 16th Edition, Saunders

Burg, Ingelfinger, Wald, Gellis & Kagan's "Current Pediatric Therapy" 14, Harcourt Brace International Edition, Saunders

Behrman, Vaughan, "Nelson Textbook of Pediatrics" 12th Edition, Saunders

0-595-31519-4